HOW TO COPE WITH DIFFICULT PARENTS

WINDY DRYDEN was born in London in 1950. He has worked in psychotherapy and counselling for over 20 years and is the author or editor of more than 85 books, including *The Incredible Sulk* (1992), *Overcoming Guilt* (1994) and *Ten Steps to Positive Living* (1994). Dr Dryden is Professor of Counselling at Goldsmiths College, University of London.

Born in Dundee, Scotland, JACK GORDON is a graduate member of the British Psychological Society. He trained in Rational Emotive Behaviour Therapy under Professor Dryden and devotes his time to counselling and writing on REBT.

Windy Dryden and Jack Gordon are also the authors of *Think Your Way to Happiness, How to Untangle Your Emotional Knots, Beating the Comfort Trap* and *How to Cope When the Going gets Tough* (Sheldon Press 1990, 1991, 1993, and 1994).

Overcoming Common Problems Series

For a full list of titles please contact
Sheldon Press, Marylebone Road, London NW1 4DU

The Assestiveness Workbook
A plan for busy women
JOANNA GUTMANN

Birth Over Thirty
SHEILA KITZINGER

Body Language
How to read others' thoughts by their
gestures
ALLAN PEASE

Body Language in Relationships
DAVID COHEN

Calm Down
How to cope with frustration and anger
DR PAUL HAUCK

Changing Course
How to take charge of your career
SUE DYSON AND STEPHEN HOARE

Comfort for Depression
JANET HORWOOD

Coping Successfully with Agoraphobia
DR KENNETH HAMBLY

Coping Successfully with Migraine
SUE DYSON

Coping Successfully with Pain
NEVILLE SHONE

Coping Successfully with Panic Attacks
SHIRLEY TRICKETT

Coping Successfully with Prostate Problems
ROSY REYNOLDS

Coping Successfully with Your Hyperactive Child
DR PAUL CARSON

Coping Successfully with Your Irritable Bowel
ROSEMARY NICOL

Coping Successfully with Your Second Child
FIONA MARSHALL

Coping with Anxiety and Depression
SHIRLEY TRICKETT

Coping with Blushing
DR ROBERT EDELMANN

Coping with Cot Death
SARAH MURPHY

Coping with Depression and Elation
DR PATRICK McKEON

Coping with Strokes
DR TOM SMITH

Coping with Suicide
DR DONALD SCOTT

Coping with Thrush
CAROLINE CLAYTON

Curing Arthritis – The Drug-Free Way
MARGARET HILLS

Curing Arthritis
More ways to a drug-free life
MARGARET HILLS

Curing Arthritis Diet Book
MARGARET HILLS

Curing Coughs, Colds and Flu – The Drug-Free Way
MARGARET HILLS

Curing Illness – The Drug-Free Way
MARGARET HILLS

Depression
DR PAUL HAUCK

Divorce and Separation
Every woman's guide to a new life
ANGELA WILLIAMS

Don't Blame Me!
How to stop blaming yourself and other people
TONY GOUGH

Everything You Need to Know about Shingles
DR ROBERT YOUNGSON

Family First Aid and Emergency Handbook
DR ANDREW SRANWAY

Overcoming Common Problems Series

Fight Your Phobia and Win
DAVID LEWIS

Getting Along with People
DIANNE DOUBTFIRE

Getting Married
JOANNA MOORHEAD

Getting the Best for your Bad Back
DR ANTHONY CAMPBELL

Goodbye Backache
DR DAVID IMRIE WITH COLLEEN DIMSON

Heart Attacks – Prevent and Survive
DR TOM SMITH

Helping Children Cope with Divorce
ROSEMARY WELLS

Helping Children Cope with Grief
ROSEMARY WELLS

Helping Children Cope with Stress
URSULA MARKHAM

Hold Your Head Up High
DR PAUL HAUCK

How to Be Your Own Best Friend
DR PAUL HAUCK

How to Cope with Splitting Up
VERA PEIFFER

How to Cope with Stress
DR PETER TYRER

How to Cope with Tinnltus and Hearing Loss
DR ROBERT YOUNGSON

How to Do What You Want to Do
DR PAUL HAUCK

How to Improve Your Confidence
DR KENNETH HAMBLY

How to Interview and Be Interviewed
MICHELE BROWN AND GYLES
BRANDRETH

How to Love and be Loved
DR PAUL HAUCK

How to Negotiate Successfully
PATRICK FORSYTH

How to Pass Your Driving Test
DONALD RIDLAND

How to Solve Your Problems
BRENDA ROGERS

How to Spot Your Child's Potential
CECILE DROUIN AND ALAIN DUBOS

How to Stand Up for Yourself
DR PAUL HAUCK

How to Start a Conversation and Make Friends
DON GABOR

How to Stop Worrying
DR FRANK TALLIS

How to Survive Your Teenagers
SHELIA DAINOW

How to Untangle Your Emotional Knots
DR WINDY DRYDEN AND JACK GORDON

Hysterectomy
SUZIE HAYMAN

Is HRT Right for You?
DR ANNE MACGREGOR

The Incredible Sulk
DR WINDY DRYDEN

The Irritable Bowel Diet Book
ROSEMARY NICOL

The Irritable Bowel Stress Book
ROSEMARY NICOL

Jealousy
DR PAUL HAUCK

Learning from Experience
A woman's guide to getting older without panic
PATRICIA O'BRIEN

Learning to Live with Multiple Sclerosis
DR ROBERT POVEY, ROBIN DOWIE AND
GILLIAN PRETT

Living Through Personal Crisis
ANN KAISER STEARNS

Living with Grief
DR TONY LAKE

Overcoming Common Problems Series

Overcoming Common Problems

HOW TO COPE WITH DIFFICULT PARENTS

Dr Windy Dryden
and Jack Gordon

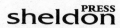

First published in Great Britain in 1995 by
Sheldon Press, SPCK, Marylebone Road, London NW1 4DU

British Library Cataloguing-in-Publication Data
A catalogue record for this book is available from the British Library

ISBN 0–85969–738–X

Photoset by Deltatype Ltd, Ellesmere Port, Cheshire
Printed in Great Britain by Biddles Ltd, Guildford and King's Lynn

Contents

Introduction

Quite a few books have appeared over the past two or three years with advice to young – and not so young – adults on how to get on better with their parents, or how to make peace with their parents, or even how to overcome the traumas of having been brought up in a troubled family. So, why another book on how to cope with parents who treat you in ways that you find difficult to understand and deal with? Are we dissatisfied with the quality of advice you will find in these other books? No, not necessarily. Much of the advice offered you looks good in print; you'll find good sensible, practical advice on better ways of communicating with your parents, learning how to express your feelings towards them in more appropriate ways – all good stuff that could potentially be helpful to you *if you knew how to use it.* There's the rub: good advice can be useful, but even the best advice in the world won't do you much good if you don't know how to apply it to get the results you want. You may read, for example, that good communication between you and your parents depends on what shape your relationship is in. The closer the relationship, the easier it will be to communicate with them. OK? Then you will read that building a closer relationship depends on better ways of communicating your feelings. But if your relationship with your parents is already in a pretty tacky state, and the quality of your 'communication' next to zero, what do you do? You will feel you are in a catch-22 situation: which comes first? It's like chasing your tail.

This is where this book makes the difference. We wrote it because we have something special to offer you. We know the kind of problems you experience with 'difficult' parents because we counsel people with similar problems practically every day in our professional lives. We understand how you feel about parents who are over-critical, or over-demanding or over-dependent, and we know the obstacles you face when you try to communicate what is bothering you as you seek practical solutions to your problems.

The good news is that help is at hand! The kind of problems parents can cause you in adult life are not insurmountable; you can learn how to resolve them by means of a special approach we will teach you that goes to the very roots of these problems. It is this new approach that is one of the keys that makes this book special. As you learn how to use it

1

you will come to see that it provides you with a framework for understanding and resolving virtually any emotional difficulty you may experience with 'difficult' parents. In short, we'll show you how to 'get through' to your parents, to communicate effectively with them; at the same time you learn how to reduce your own frustration and emotional overreactions.

If you have read any of our previous books published by Sheldon Press you will be no stranger to our approach to dealing with personal and relationship problems. On the other hand, if you are new to our ideas, welcome! You are about to be presented with a system of ideas and methods researched, developed and tested by many mental health practitioners around the world. It has been shown to be unusually effective in helping people to overcome the kind of problems you will meet in this book. You may find our approach new, even exciting, but above all it is designed to be helpful.

The reason we need a new approach to resolving the kind of problems that arise between parents and their adult offspring today is not because the problems themselves are new. The problems were around in your parents' days, even your grandparents' days. What *is* new is that today our values have changed, our expectations have changed and our perceived obligations, both to ourselves and to our parents, have changed. That is why we need a whole new approach to the way we think about ourselves and our relationship with our parents. So, if you are ready to begin your journey of discovery, let's go.

We believe that, generally speaking, parents and their adult offspring *want* to get on with each other and to maintain a reasonably happy relationship throughout most of their lives together. Unfortunately, these normal, healthy desires are frequently thwarted by mutual misunderstandings, unrealistic expectations and demands. Potentially amicable relations between you and your parents become instead arenas of acrimony and conflict. Our aim in this book is to show you how to avoid such undesirable outcomes and to offer you practical, effective methods of bringing about a mutually acceptable relationship with your parents, even if relations between you at the moment are in fairly poor shape.

As the authors of this book, we have accumulated between us a considerable amount of theoretical knowledge and many thousands of hours of working experience in helping people to overcome their personal and relationship problems. If you read this book carefully and carry out the Three Key Tasks in the order in which they are presented, you should find yourself in a much stronger position to live your life the way you want to live it *and* to get on better with your 'difficult' parents, irrespective of whether you were brought up by two parents, one parent, or a parent substitute. If that is your goal, you have already taken your first steps to achieving it by picking up this book.

Let us offer you a brief foretaste of what is to come. Right from the start you will learn through typical case histories how to structure the kind of problem you might be having with your parents around three interrelated Key Tasks. You will be getting involved quite soon with these vitally important Tasks. So let us briefly introduce them: *Key Task No. 1: Getting Yourself into a Healthy Frame of Mind Emotionally* provides you with a model and a set of practical procedures to enable you to see your situation vis-à-vis your parents in a new light. You will learn how to remove the emotional 'clutter' and unconstructive negative attitudes that hold you back and interfere with your ability to understand and resolve the kind of problems you typically experience when trying to cope with 'difficult' parents.

For example, are your parents constantly criticizing you and picking faults? Nothing you do is right? You are always being told that you should do this, or not do that? And when you cut short the time you spend with them to escape from the continual nagging, or even lose your temper and angrily argue back and try to justify your lifestyle, they accuse you of not listening, or even not loving them any more? Sounds familiar?

Or, have your parents made it clear to you that they feel very hurt because you have left the parental home to live independently on your own, and although you believe you are doing the right thing, you still feel guilty about 'hurting' them? Or perhaps you feel guilty because you realise you don't love them any more?

If you are feeling angry or guilty or in some other way you are emotionally overreacting to the way your parents are treating you, these negative attitudes will block any attempts you might make to try to improve your relationship with them. Your parents feel upset, let us suppose, over the way they see you behaving. But if *you* feel emotionally upset over the way *they* are reacting, then the chances are that neither of you will be able even to discuss your differences in a rational manner. *Key Task No. 1* is designed to help you to unchain your mind. It shows you how to remove those emotional roadblocks to effective communication and shows you how to develop more rational and constructive attitudes as a foundation to accomplishing your

3

second Key Task.

Key Task No. 2: Understanding and Accepting Your Parents with their Difficult Traits and Behaviour is basically about *what* you need to know to get on better terms with your parents. We explain what it means to understand and accept your parents and why it is important to do so if you wish to get along with them more amicably. By means of practical examples or case histories that most people can relate to, we show you *how* to translate your new knowledge into action. You will also learn how to acquire a number of skills that can help you to bring about a better mutual understanding of your respective viewpoints and to accept that both you and your parents have the right to differ on, but need not fight over, issues that cannot, for the moment, be resolved. Next we focus on your third Key Task.

Key Task No. 3: Acting In An Enlightened Self-Interested Way Towards Your Parents means taking responsibility for your own life. Here we pinpoint the importance of pursuing your own life goals and purposes and striving primarily for your own happiness, while acknowledging that your parents have an equal right to strive for what they regard as important to them. We distinguish self-interest from selfishness and discuss the issue of sacrificing your own vital interests for your parents' sake. We offer guidelines on striking a sensible balance by deciding when, how far, and in what circumstances such self-sacrifice on your part may be justifiable.

The six chapters in this book cover a range of problems typical of those that parents can cause their children in adult life. Each chapter is built around the Three Key Tasks and outlines methods, illustrated by practical examples, of combating the internal blocks to effective communication such as anxiety, anger or guilt, together with practical methods of increasing your ability to communicate more effectively in your relationship with your parents.

We briefly considered including a chapter on coping with parents who are abusive, an issue that has recently attracted much publicity. However, abuse of children is a complex issue that would justify a book to itself to do it justice. Moreover, since the victims of childhood physical and/or sexual abuse often require professional help in later life to cope with the after-effects of their earlier experiences, we decided that a brief discussion of the subject would serve no useful purpose.

Finally, an afterword concludes the book with a summary of the key points and insights throughout the text and adds a few useful tips on how to derive the maximum benefit from your reading of the book. If you want to make an unsatisfactory relationship with your parents truly a thing of the past, as well as discover your potential for leading a happier, more fulfilling existence, make a start now with this book!

1

The Three Tasks in Coping
with Difficult Parents

Adult offspring often find it hard to cope with parents who are in some way 'difficult'. This is not something new, of course; inter-generational conflict has been around in some form or another for a long time. Parents can be neglectful, rejecting, demanding, dictatorial, over-critical, abusive or out of touch with modern life, to name but a few ways in which they can make life difficult for their adult offspring as well as for themselves. We are not saying that 'difficult' parents are necessarily only, or always, 'difficult'; more accurately, it is that they tend to behave in ways that sometimes (or often) make life difficult for their grown-up children or adult offspring.

What is new, though, is the fact that the problem of difficult parents is becoming more widespread! The demographic data show that the over-65s are one of the fastest growing age groups in the Western world, for improved health care means that people are living longer on average than they did seventy or so years ago. This increased longevity, coupled with the tendency towards early marriage and childbirth among younger people, has created a bigger overlap between the generations. It is not unusual to find grandparents who are only in their forties, and great-grandparents in their sixties.

A consequence of the failure to overcome patterns of behaviour that create difficulties between people of different generations, such as adult children and their parents, is that communication deteriorates – and sometimes even breaks down completely – leaving both parties feeling misunderstood, bitter and alienated.

Our aim in this chapter is to introduce you to the 'Three Key Tasks' that need to be memorized and put into practice if you wish to learn how to cope successfully with 'difficult' parents. These Key Tasks are:

1. Getting yourself into a healthy frame of mind emotionally.
2. Understanding and accepting your parents with their difficult traits and behaviour.
3. Acting in an enlightened self-interested way towards your parents.

Our aim is not so much to restore those feelings of love that you and your parents may once have shared (although that outcome is possible, and would be a definite bonus for all concerned if it happened); instead, and more realistically, we hope to show you how you can act in such a way as to minimize (but not, unfortunately, eradicate) conflict with difficult parents. We aim to help you to a better understanding of both your own feelings and those of your parents, so that you can make optimum use of your natural problem-solving abilities to recover from past traumas and present negative experiences (and even put them to your advantage). Once you achieve that, the road may then be open for you to pursue ways of rebuilding your relationship with your parents, with the focus upon the development of mutual understanding, affection and respect. A further bonus of achieving a true awareness and acceptance of your difficult parents, plus the ability to cope with them, is that the knowledge and experience you will gain may well stand you in good stead should you one day become a difficult parent yourself!

Your Three Key Tasks

The Three Key Tasks that we will now present and explain to you form the keystone around which the rest of this book is structured. It is therefore important that you understand and practise these if you want to learn how to cope with your difficult parents.

Key Task No. 1: Getting yourself into a healthy frame of mind emotionally

It needs to be made clear that this does not mean getting yourself into a 'good mood'. Some people believe in waiting until they feel 'in the mood' before they tackle some difficult task. Yet waiting until you are 'in the mood' before you do something that needs to be done now can often mean waiting a very long time indeed! In fact, we're not talking about 'moods' here. Let's face it, if you feel angry and resentful towards one or both of your parents, if you think you are put down and victimized by their actions and the way they are treating you now or have treated you in the past, and if you blame them continually for being the way they were and still are, you are unlikely to make any headway towards improving matters by waiting for your 'mood' to change. Blame tends to beget blame; and expressed anger can lead to a shouting match, hurt feelings and sullen withdrawal and sulking. Before long, you find that you and your parents are no longer in communication.

However exasperating your parents' attitudes towards you may be (and there will be times when you feel their attitudes or actions are driving you crazy), you need to realize that it is not your parents' behaviour that is causing your emotional distress – it is *the way you view it* that is the problem. Granted, you wouldn't feel angry and resentful towards your parents if they were treating you well, and their difficult behaviour certainly contributes to your negative upset feelings. But their behaviour doesn't *cause* your upset feelings. If, for example, your parents told you that they didn't want to see you ever again, you might react in a variety of ways. Some people would feel very upset, others would feel sad or disappointed, while yet others might shrug their shoulders and forget about it.

So what accounts for these very different reactions to the same event? The answer is that other people's words or actions don't *make* us angry or emotionally disturbed, but that we create our own feelings about the situation via the way we think about and evaluate what is happening to us. Let's take a moment to convince you of the truth of this seemingly odd (but nevertheless very important) insight.

You feel as you think

'You feel as you think' summarizes an important insight, which we shall call REBT Insight No. 1. REBT stands for Rational Emotive Behaviour Therapy, an innovative research-tested system of psychological counselling and training that was originated and developed by Dr Albert Ellis, a famous clinical psycholigist in the United States. It is a system of counselling that is currently used by many practitioners (including ourselves) throughout the world, with very impressive results. For our present purposes, you can think of REBT (formerly known as RET) as a practical, action-oriented approach to help you to reduce or eliminate common emotional problems (such as the kind of problems you might have when coping with difficult parents) and to enhance your personal growth.

You are now about to take the first steps towards developing that inner psychological strength – that 'emotional muscle' – you will need to cope successfully with difficult parents.

Like all muscle development, you will need to practise the exercises! Don't worry, they're not difficult. The more you work at them, though, the more confident you will become at using them.

So let's begin with REBT Insight No. 1:

REBT Insight No. 1

You feel as you think, and all your thoughts, feelings and behaviour are interrelated.

Many experiments conducted over the past few years have shown that human emotions do not magically exist in their own right, but almost always stem from ideas, beliefs or attitudes that can usually be changed by modifying one's thinking processes. In other words, if you change the way you think, you also tend to change the way you feel – and the way you subsequently act or behave. If feelings stem directly from our attitudes or beliefs, it follows that common emotional problems like anxiety, depression, guilt, self-hatred and anger stem not from what happens to us, but from our *attitudes* about what happens to us. That is the meaning of 'you feel as you think'.

The A–B–C model of emotional disturbance

In this section, we present the A–B–C model of emotional disturbance:

A stands for *Activating Event* (for example, some unpleasant or unwanted happening, such as being rejected or severely criticized, or the prospect of facing a similar stressful event in the near future).

B stands for your *Belief System* – in other words, your thoughts and attitudes about what is happening to you. **B** comprises the ways in which you habitually think about and evaluate events in your life. There are basically two kinds of beliefs:Rational *beliefs* and irrational *beliefs*. These are known as rBs and iBs respectively, and will generally be used in their abbreviated form in the subsequent text.

C stands for the emotional and behavioural *Consequences* you experience as a result of the beliefs you hold about **A**. Your emotional Consequences, or feelings, can be divided into two types: healthy and unhealthy. And as your thoughts, feelings and behaviour are, as previously emphasized, interrelated, your behavioural Consequences, or actions, also fit basically into two categories: constructive and unconstructive.

The points to note here are:

A does *not* cause C.
A is first perceived, and then evaluated by B.

C then responds to and reflects the kind of beliefs held at **B** about what is happening at **A**.

You have now been introduced to the A–B–C model of emotional disturbance, an explanatory device used extensively in REBT. When you feel confident that you fully understand the A–B–C model, you can proceed with us to the next stage.

Two kinds of thinking, feeling and behaviour

In the explanation of the A–B–C model, we made reference to rational beliefs (rBs) and irrational beliefs (iBs), to healthy and unhealthy feelings, and to constructive and unconstructive acts or behaviours. As you may have suspected, there is a very important connection between these three pairs. You will recall that we stated that thinking, feeling and behaving are all interrelated; if you change one, you tend to see changes in the other two. We can now state the following basic principles:

Rational beliefs (rBs) lead to healthy emotions and to constructive action and behaviour;
Irrational beliefs (iBs) lead to unhealthy (disturbed) emotions and to unconstructive action and behaviour.

Thinking and self-awareness are products of human consciousness, as are feelings and behaviour, but it is mainly through thinking that we make decisions to guide our actions and behaviour to survive and to get what we want in life. Thus, if we wish to change the way we feel and behave, we need to change the way we think. You will see presently that it is more efficient to change thinking first, and *then* reinforce and deepen these changes with a variety of behavioural techniques.

If you have followed us so far, you will want to know how to distinguish rBs from iBs, and so we turn our attention now to this issue – which is the whole crux of getting yourself into a healthy frame of mind emotionally, which in turn is a prerequisite for coping with difficult parents and other potentially stressful situations. Once you can distinguish rBs from iBs, you will then be able to see why the former lead to healthy emotions and constructive behaviour, while the latter do not.

Goals, purposes and rationality

All of us have preferences, wants and wishes in life, and we seem to be at our happiest when we set up important life goals and actively strive to achieve them. So long as we succeed in getting what we want, we usually feel happy and contented. But when – as will almost certainly happen from time to time – we are blocked from getting our desires fulfilled, we experience negative emotions. Whether these are healthy or unhealthy depends upon the way we view things when our desires are not met. REBT defines our attitudes or beliefs as rational, our feelings as healthy, and our behaviour as constructive, if these attributes are helping us to achieve our basic goals.

Conversely, if our attitudes, feelings and behaviour hinder the pursuit of our basic goals, they are deemed irrational, unhealthy and unconstructive respectively. Both rational and irrational philosophies can be identified and distinguished by four main characteristics, as shown in Table 1. You should study this table carefully, as you will need to understand correctly the features that distinguish rational statements from irrational statements as you proceed through this book.

Table 1   Distinguishing features of rationality and irrationality

Rationality	Irrationality
Consists of wants, wishes and preferences.	Consists of unqualified demands, commands and dictates.
Is logical, and aids effective decision-making	Is illogical, and fosters magical thinking.
Is consistent with reality, encourages us to deal with things as they are, and to attempt to change them if they can be changed.	Is inconsistent with reality, and discourages us from dealing with things as they are.
Leads to healthy emotions, and aids constructive action.	Leads to poor results for us emotionally and behaviourally.

With the information we now have, we can go straight into an example of how to use the A–B–C model of emotional disturbance.

Since understanding the model is of key importance to you if you wish to derive practical benefit from this book, we have used an example of a man who is having difficulty in getting on with his father in order to help you see the model in action. This is a typical experience that many readers will be able to relate to, and will help to clarify the model.

Using the A–B–C model of emotional disturbance

Gary was a 40-year-old company executive who had great difficulty in getting on with his father. The trouble was, as Gary explained, 'My father is always criticizing me. Nothing I can do or say is right. If he isn't on about my choice of friends, or making sarcastic comments about my choice in clothes, he tells me how I'm only wasting my money on the things I buy, that I've got no money sense, and that if he had had the chances that I had when he was my age, he would have got himself a far better job than the one I have now. I suppose he means well – he says that he loves me, and that his criticisms are for my own good – but there are times when I could kill him for treating me as if I was still a child!'

Gary did not mean the last sentence literally, of course. In fact, he said that he loved his father, but felt he had to keep a tight lid on his conflicting feelings. So far, Gary had managed to avoid a direct confrontation with his father during their strained conversations. Their meetings would last only an hour or two; but as soon as his father had left, Gary's resentment would explode – and in no time at all he would be found down at the pub on a drinking binge.

As we've already pointed out, the A–B–C model is an explanatory device to help us understand how common emotional problems are determined not by unpleasant experiences, but by the attitudes we adopt towards these experiences. So let's take Gary's problems as an example. Some of you may have inferred that Gary's problem goes right back to his childhood, when he was probably subjected to a lot of criticism and bullying from his father, and that now, in later life, Gary is simply hanging on to old resentments and re-enacting old quarrels with his father. Your assessment may be correct; Gary may well have *always* had difficulty in relating to his father. However, we can't change the past, and besides, what we are really interested in is not finding out how Gary originally acquired his problem with his father, but why Gary is *still* carrying this resentment towards his father today – when he is no longer a boy in his father's care, but an adult in his own right. So let's see if what we know so far can provide us with an answer to our question.

The A–B–C of Gary's anger towards his father

At point **A**, the Activating Event, Gary's father is criticizing aspects of Gary's life in a way that would be more appropriate for an adult lecturing a child. At point **C**, the emotional Consequence, Gary is seething with resentment at having his lifestyle continually criticized and being spoken to as if he was still a child.

Now we know that Gary finds that he cannot manage his anger; for every time his father visits him, Gary ends up with resentment that he tries to anaesthetize with liberal doses of alcohol. Gary still has his anger problem, and if he continues to try to quell the pain by drinking, he is likely to wind up with even more painful health consequences later. Thus Gary's reactions to his father's criticisms are obviously self-defeating. They will do nothing to help Gary to get on better with his father, which is what he would like, and these sessions with his father in which Gary is suppressing his anger in order to avoid an angry confrontation may ultimately harm his health.

REBT states that we can discover the nature of someone's Belief System (point **B**) by knowing the facts at **A** and **C**. People have only a relatively limited number of emotions they can experience, and these emotions fall under a few major headings. We know too that certain thoughts or beliefs connect with certain emotions. At point **B**, what is Gary telling himself to bring on his angry feelings and self-defeating behaviour?

Gary's iBs

The following is probably a fair summary of what Gary believes about his situation:

- 'My father must not unfairly criticize me!'
- 'It's awful that he still treats me as if I was still a child!'
- 'I can't stand his treating me in such an unjust manner!'
- 'My father is a bad person who doesn't deserve to be treated with any respect whatever!'

If you refer now to Table 1 on page 12, you will see that each of Gary's beliefs about his father's constant criticism carry one or more of the distinguishing features of irrationality. That is to say, they consist of absolutist demands or dictates; they are illogical, inconsistent with reality, and lead to poor results for Gary, both emotionally and behaviourally. Since Gary's irrational convictions are producing nothing but poor results for him emotionally and are causing him to act in ways that are more likely to block, rather than enhance, the possibility of a reconciliation with his critical father, it seems sensible for Gary to give up his irrational ideas and replace them with more rational, more constructive, attitudes. How would he achieve this?

Disputing iBs

The answer is by adopting a scientific method of challenging his beliefs to discover if they hold any validity – by asking questions of them such as: 'Where is the evidence that this idea or belief of mine is correct?' 'Does this belief make logical sense?' 'Is it realistic in the sense of according with the facts?' 'Where is the evidence that would support this belief?' 'Will this belief help me to achieve my goals?' That is the method we use in REBT of challenging one's beliefs; it is called 'Disputing'. Hence, we now add **D** for Disputing to the A–B–C model.

So, to summarize, here are three criteria by which you can determine the validity of a belief:

- Is it logical?
- Is this belief consistent with reality?
- Will this belief help me to achieve my goals?

Thus in the example above of Gary's beliefs concerning the way his father treated him, you would 'Dispute' each of these beliefs as follows:

Disputing Gary's iBs
Let's take each of Gary's beliefs and question them:

- 'My father must not unfairly criticize me!' Now we apply the first of three challenges:

(a) *Is this belief logical?* Here Gary is saying that because he would very much like his father to stop his continual criticizing, therefore he absolutely has to. Does it logically follow that because you want something, your wish absolutely must be granted? Obviously not!

(b) *Is this belief consistent with reality?* Well, if it was consistent with reality, wouldn't whatever you demanded automatically be granted? If something you demand absolutely has to occur, then it would! Yet there is no law of the universe that we are aware of that gives us, or anybody else, this power. Since neither you nor we control the universe, there is no guarantee that anything you want has to be granted. Therefore the statement is not realistic. It is not in accord with reality.

(c) *Will this belief help Gary to achieve his goals?* It's very unlikely! Suppose Gary confronts his father and says, 'Look here! I'm heartily sick and tired of your continual criticism of me. You absolutely must stop it right now, do you hear me? If you don't stop, you are just a rotten person who doesn't deserve even a shred of respect ever again!' How would you expect Gary's father to react to that? Would he respond with, 'My dear boy, you are absolutely right. How could I have been so blind all these years that I failed to see what an admirable person you really are!' We very much doubt it! Gary's father would be more likely to tell Gary very angrily where to go, and slam the door behind him on his way out of the house – and out of Gary's life. Demanding that someone do as you bid may work for a time with children, but with adults – especially family – it hardly ever does.

Now let's examine the second of Gary's beliefs about the way his father is treating him:

- 'It's awful that he still treats me as if I was still a child!'

(a) *Is this belief logical?* No. We would grant that being continually criticized is bad, and most people would agree with this. However, jumping from 'bad' to 'awful' is illogical, because 'awful' doesn't mean just very bad, or even 100 per cent bad. It means 101 per cent bad, more than totally bad. So it makes no logical sense to claim that because something is bad, therefore it is more than totally bad.

(b) *Is this belief consistent with reality?* No. Nothing can be more than 100 per cent bad. Moreover, 'awful' implies that something shouldn't be as bad as it is. That is absurd, because if the conditions exist to make something bad, then it should be bad, because it is bad. It makes no sense to claim that it shouldn't be bad when it undoubtedly is bad.

(c) *Will this belief help Gary to achieve his goals?* If you convince yourself that something that is happening to you is awful, i.e. that it is worse than anything else you could ever experience or imagine, how will that motivate you to try to change the situation? You would be more likely to view your situation as hopeless, beyond any possibility of you being able to change it. That is what 'awful' really means, and since nothing can be more than 100 per cent bad, it is a term with no real meaning. Give up your 'awfulizing', and you will more likely be able to see things in perspective, especially the tragic, unpleasant and unfortunate events in your life.

Gary's third belief is very commonly held, but as you will see in a moment, it is simply untrue:

- 'I can't stand his treating me in such an unjust manner!'

(a) *Is this belief logical?* Not at all! Something may be unjust or unpleasant, but it hardly follows that being unjust or unpleasant makes it unbearable!

(b) *Is this belief consistent with reality?* In no way! If you really couldn't stand something, you would collapse and die. If you think about it, you can stand *anything* until you physically expire. Since Gary did not collapse and die, he obviously could stand that which he claimed he could not stand.

Moreover, when Gary tells himself, 'I can't stand his treating me in such an unjust manner!' he is also implying, 'And I can never have any happiness again!' Now, is there any evidence that Gary can never have any happiness again? Of course not! He would have to know his entire future in order to prove any statement made in the present about his future personal happiness. Since nobody knows what the future will bring, Gary's belief is not consistent with reality.

(c) *Will this belief help Gary to achieve his goals?* Not if Gary continues to believe that being criticized by his father is something he cannot possibly stand. If you share the irrational conviction that you can't stand someone's disagreeable behaviour, whatever it may be, you will prevent yourself from getting into the frame of mind that would enable you to view the situation as a problem to be discussed and resolved. Consequently, the problem situation is likely to continue, and perhaps even become worse.

Gary's concluding belief is:

- 'My father is a bad person who doesn't deserve to be treated with any respect whatever!'

(a) *Is this belief logical?* Gary's conclusion that his father is a bad person does not follow logically from the fact that his father criticizes

Gary. In fact, Gary's conclusion is a huge exaggeration, for Gary is singling out one aspect of his father's behaviour he considers bad, and then making a magical jump to concluding that his father's entire personhood is no good.

(b) *Is this belief consistent with reality?* Gary's error here is that he identifies the person with that person's behaviour, which is a gross over-generalization. Also, to call anyone a bad person is an arbitrary definition. Philosophically speaking, you cannot legitimately label anyone as 'good' or 'bad' on the basis of possessing some trait. You may evaluate a person's acts, deeds, character traits, beliefs and so on as good, bad or neutral, according to some external standard, or according to that person's own goals and values; but acts, deeds, performances and traits are only *aspects* of the person, never the totality. A human being is continually changing, and therefore cannot be legitimately rated in any global or once-and-for-all manner.

Lastly, calling someone a bad person and undeserving of any respect whatever is to imply that the person has some essence of badness, and that they could only and always do bad things. That, of course, is a quite unprovable statement.

(c) *Will this belief help Gary to achieve his goals?* Damning his father as a bad person who could never merit any respect is unlikely to endear Gary to his father. The pair of them are more likely to have a bust-up than to sit down and discuss ways of reaching some kind of settlement of Gary's grievances. You can take it that, generally speaking, damning someone for behaving in a way you find unacceptable will make it less likely, rather than more likely, that your demands will be met.

We have used the example of Gary's irrational attitude towards his over-critical father to emphasize the point that so long as you maintain and display irrational attitudes towards parents or parental figures who are behaving towards you in ways that make communication difficult, you will sidetrack yourself from dealing constructively with the issue of how to make your peace with one another.

We now turn our attention to the kind of beliefs and attitudes you *would* find helpful in dealing with parents who are difficult to get on with in some way; we call such beliefs 'rational alternative beliefs'. Once more, we shall take Gary as an example.

Gary's rational alternative beliefs

Once Gary had truly convinced himself that his attitudes towards his father were irrational, emotionally upsetting and driving him into a no-win situation, what rational alternative beliefs could Gary develop that would lessen his emotional tension and encourage him to try out ways of communicating his concerns to his father in ways that might lead to better mutual understanding and acceptance? We would suggest that Gary could come up with something along these lines:

- 'I would strongly prefer my father to become a lot less critical of me and my lifestyle, but he doesn't have to.'

- 'It's a pain in the neck when he goes on and on and talks to me as if I was still a youngster, but it isn't awful. It's just the way he is at the present time. Maybe if I learn to listen and let him see that I understand his point of view, I may be able to get him to see my point of view without having to agree with it.'

- 'If he doesn't change, I'll never like being treated like a child, but I can definitely stand it. I can still accept him as he is without convincing myself that it's unbearable.'

- 'My father is a fallible human being like the rest of us, who may be set in his ways, and who possibly doesn't know how to change, or doesn't want to. He doesn't *have* to change. He is entitled to hold whatever views he wants to without being condemned for them. It would be nice if he could be persuaded to be less critical, but even if he can't be, there is no reason why his right to express his views cannot be respected even if we continue to disagree on most of them.'

If Gary could replace his previous irrational convictions with these more rational ones, how would he feel? He would feel annoyed, disappointed – and possibly a little sad – if his father continued to criticize him unnecessarily, but he would not feel angry and resentful towards his father. Instead, Gary would try various ways of showing his father that while he could not go along with his father's criticisms, he accepted his father as a fallible human being who has the right to his views. Gary could even explain to his father that if he, Gary, had been brought up the way his father had been brought up and had lived through the experiences his father had gone through, he might well see things in the same way as his father does today. Freed from the necessity to prove himself right and his father wrong, Gary could be more sympathetic towards his father; and without surrendering his

19

own convictions about how to live his own life, Gary would work at helping his father to see that a father and son can learn to accept each other with their respective differences, and still maintain an affectionate relationship.

We have devoted the bulk of this chapter to explaining how strongly held iBs and attitudes, and the self-defeating emotions and behaviours that spring from them, can sabotage one's efforts to cope successfully with difficult parents. You have been shown how to identify these iBs from the absolutistic forms they take, and you have been shown the techniques for Disputing some typical iBs in a way that will help you to recognize your own iBs and replace them with more rational alternatives.

As you proceed through this book, you will gain several more insights and also learn some very useful methods to strengthen your 'psychological muscle' for accomplishing the tasks that lie ahead. However, before moving on to discuss the remaining two Key Tasks, we will offer you one more important insight into emotional disturbance.

Letting go of the past

Perhaps most of the difficulties that adults experience in relating to their parents stem from highly charged emotional incidents that such adult offspring experienced in their childhood relationship with their parents. Unresolved conflicts tend to live on, and you may believe that certain things your parents did or said to you when you were a child 'made' you feel hurt and resentful. You may even believe that those early painful memories are the cause of your difficulties in relating to your parents today.

As a child you tended to believe and do what you were told. If you were sometimes ignored, belittled, manipulated or psychologically attacked in some other way, you suffered because you did not know how to deal with these attacks. But today, you *do* know! REBT Insight No.1 explained how the emotional problems and tensions you experienced when you were young were not caused by what your parents did to you, but by the way you viewed and reacted to what your parents did. You know, too, that you don't have to re-run those painful early psychological memories in order to wipe them out. You may well feel better by re-living and expressing these painful emotions – the anger, the buried resentment, the fear – associated with your early traumas, but in order to *get* better, to be able to let go of those painful feelings and self-defeating behaviour patterns that still bedevil you today, you need to rid yourself of the iBs you originally held about the unfortunate things that happened to you in the past.

In other words, it is less a question of facing up to these emotionally charged childhood incidents, and releasing the powerful feelings associated with them, but rather of focusing upon the attitudes you brought to bear upon these childhood incidents – attitudes that you *still* are carrying around inside you, consciously or subconsciously. If you want to rid yourself of your unhealthy emotions about the past, then you have to change your attitudes about your early traumas. Our attitudes about the past can sabotage our ability to cope with parents who, in some way, are being difficult in the present. This brings us to REBT Insight No. 2, which is printed in the box below. You will see that it follows logically from REBT Insight No. 1, which you encountered on page 10.

REBT Insight No. 2

Regardless of how you disturbed yourself in the past, you are disturbed now because you still believe the iBs with which you created your disturbed feelings in the past. Moreover, you are still reindoctrinating yourself with these unsustainable beliefs, not because you were previously 'conditioned' to hold these beliefs and now do so 'automatically', but because you are continually reinforcing these ideas by your present inappropriate actions or inaction, in addition to your unrealistic thinking.

In other words, it is people's current thinking that maintains their disturbed emotions and behaviour, and enables these to hold sway over their life in the present. Now let's go on to introduce you to your second Key Task.

Key Task No. 2: Understanding and accepting your parents with their difficult traits and behaviour

This is the second of the Three Key Tasks that you will need to practise when coping with difficult parents.

Since your present task is to learn how to understand and accept a difficult parent or parents, you may find it helpful to bear in mind that, fundamentally, there are three main reasons for parents' difficult behaviour:

(i) *Ignorance*   Parents may be unaware of certain facts that are common knowledge to their adult offspring, or they may lack up-to-date information about the world they live in of the kind that the younger generation takes for granted. Being out of touch with what's going on can lead to communication difficulties between adult children and their parents.

(ii) *Emotional disturbance*   Parents who are emotionally disturbed in some way will tend to act in inappropriate ways because of their disturbed feelings. As a consequence, the adult children of such parents will need to acquire a degree of understanding of these problems, and may even wish to enlist professional help, to help them cope with their parents' disturbed behaviour.

(iii) *Deficiency*   We are talking here of parents of limited intelligence who lack the basic skills they need to understand and relate to their adult children. Also, parents suffering from various forms of physiological or psychological impairment can create difficulties for their offspring through experiencing severe failures of memory, or by acting in ways (both inside and outside the home) that can sometimes bring about potentially harmful consequences.

What it means to understand and accept parents

Difficult parents don't deliberately set out to make life difficult for you. It may be that they've always been difficult; others just become difficult as a result of ageing. For example, I (Jack Gordon) had parents who married relatively late in life and who were very set in their ways. I believe they loved me, but there were times when they had a funny way of showing it. They thought they always knew best, and they made sure that I knew it. As I grew up and learned more about what makes people tick, I could see that my parents meant well, but that they lacked up-to-date information on all sorts of things. It seemed silly to me to blame my parents because they were ignorant of certain matters; it wasn't necessarily their fault. I gradually realized that parents are, in turn, the products of their parents and their parental upbringing; and since none of us can choose our parents, the sensible thing seemed to be to try to understand one's parents, to sympathize with the difficulties they had with their own parents, and not to damn them in any way for their shortcomings.

In the light of the knowledge we have today about the genetic or biological underpinnings of human behaviour, together with our psychological and sociological insights, we are perhaps in a unique position of being able to understand our forebears in a way that they could never have understood themselves, and still less their descendants.

In the following chapters we shall invite you to examine typical kinds of behaviour shown by various types of difficult parents, and we will show you how to understand their behaviour by applying the psychological insights you will be learning as you proceed through this book. Understanding your difficult parents boils down to uncovering the beliefs, attitudes and values they've acquired over their lifetime, and that largely govern the way they behave today.

Accepting your parents means taking them as they are and refusing to condemn them for displaying traits and behaviours that you find awkward or difficult to cope with. As we argued in a previous section, your traits, deeds or performances are only aspects of you; they are never your totality. Since your acts never equal you, it follows that nobody can legitimately be rated in a once-and-for-all manner as good, bad or anything else merely on the basis of whatever characteristics they possess. As we showed you earlier, even the adjective 'difficult' is an over-generalization, for it implies that a difficult person can never be anything but difficult, has always been difficult, and always will be difficult. This is obviously untrue. Accepting people as they are with their faults and shortcomings, while endeavouring to help them, where possible, to overcome their failings, will provide a better basis for developing mutual understanding than condemning them for having failings. Understanding and acceptance go together.

Key Task No. 3: Acting in an enlightened self-interested way towards your parents

According to the philosophy of REBT, humans are happiest when we set up important life goals and actively strive to achieve them. Yet while we strive to pursue our own goals and to be happy, we need to be mindful that we live in a social world, with others who have their own goals.

Thus in dealing with our parents, enlightened self-interest means that we pursue our own goals while acknowledging that our parents have an equal right to strive for the goals that they regard as significant in their lives. As we have already suggested, unfortunately not everyone acts morally, and their unacceptable or difficult behaviour may at times be due in some measure to ignorance, emotional disturbance or some kind of deficiency. This is sometimes true also of difficult parents, who may act as if they were blind to the legitimate rights of their adult offspring, or behave in ways that deliberately disregard these rights. You will meet examples of this kind of behaviour later, with suggestions on how to deal with it. Usually, however, we believe that it is better to treat other people properly with due concern for their rights – partly because we want to be, in turn, treated properly by others, and partly because we want to help create the kind of world that it is safe and good for us to live in. Morality, when it is rational, is based to some extent on self-interested motives.

This does not mean that some degree of self-sacrifice is never justified. There can be circumstances, notably when you are caring for some loved one, such as an elderly parent, when you may legitimately put the parent's interests above your own, if you find personal meaning and happiness in doing so. However, when putting the interests of parents or others first becomes overwhelming and apparently without some end in sight, or when it is demanded of you unconditionally, we would argue that such self-sacrificing conduct is probably irrational in that it may not only be self-defeating, but may also subtly harm the person receiving the attention. Thus *excessive* self-sacrifice is discouraged here – unless of course you genuinely want to sacrifice yourself, and find personal meaning and happiness in doing so.

Clearly, enlightened self-interest is not to be confused with selfishness. Essentially, the selfish individual is out for his or her own good only, and cynically disregards the rights and wishes of others. By contrast, the individual who acts out of enlightened self-interest acts on the basis of responsible self- and social interest. He or she will put themselves first most of the time, and significant others a close second.

In the next chapter, we will show you how to cope when you don't love your parents. You may have loved them at one time, perhaps during your childhood and when you were growing up, and then later realized that you no longer loved them; or, you may never have really loved your parents. We will show you why this happens. Then, building upon the REBT Insights and the Three Key Tasks you have been introduced to in this chapter, you will see how to apply these to the possible emotional problems you may experience in this situation.

2

How to Cope when You Don't Love Your Parents

As infants, there is evidence that we are biologically programmed to be attached to our parents. Our very survival depends literally on being loved in the sense of being looked after – by our parents or parent substitutes. The English psychiatrist John Bowlby, who laid the foundation of what has become called 'attachment theory', believed that infants are born with the need for social attachments to their care-givers (usually the mother), and that this need is transferred to other individuals later in life. Certainly, a biological survival advantage is conferred upon infants who receive healthy, nourishing care through childhood and into early adulthood. As they grow older, children love their parents because they feed and clothe them, give them security, and play with them. Children's lives revolve around their parents and they often meet their offspring's deepest desires.

Even if our parents don't meet our deepest desires, we often still love them because we blame ourselves for their failures. Viewing the situation in this way is less threatening for us than concluding that our parents don't love us. Still later, as we reach adolescence and begin to relate to others, we may share activities with our parents. They take us shopping, they take us on holiday, or to sports events, etc. At this stage, bonds can develop between parents and offspring based on shared interests and activities. If asked, most offspring would reply, 'Yes, of course I love my parents.'

Leaving our childhood behind

As young adults, we outgrow our childhood dependency on our parents and develop our own interests, ideals and values. We tend to spend less and less time with our parents and elders, and more time with our peers and those who share out taste in clothes, music, entertainment, etc. Once we begin to earn a regular income, we may leave home and become completely independent of our parents. If our parents accept us and show that they understand our developing adult feelings and interests, we tend to love and respect them. In other words, we 'get on' with our parents.

Parental difficulties with 'letting go'

However, not all parents help their children to make a smooth transition to adult independence. Because of unresolved problems of their own, some parents have difficulty in letting go of their growing-up or grown-up children; these parents often want to keep their adult children at home and control their lives much as they did when their children were in their care, and were dependent upon them for everything. This leads to mutual antagonism, distrust and conflict between parents and their adult children. Instead of love and under-standing, the young adult receives only disapproval and criticism. To the young adult, those previously lovable qualities that both parents had once seemed to possess appear now to be shrivelling up before their very eyes!

When we no longer love our parents

Cultural messages and upbringing stress that we must love our parents. Hence if we no longer love our parents, but think we should, the result is often a feeling of guilt. Some parents, in an attempt to cling on to their adult children, may sometimes try to induce a feeling of guilt when they perceive that their offspring no longer love them.

To show you how to cope with parents when they try to manipulate you into doing what they want by pressing your 'guilt buttons' (that is, particular areas where you feel very vulnerable to feeling guilty), we will distinguish and explain two basically different situations:

1. Where you have never loved your parents.
2. Where you once loved your parents, but have now ceased to love them.

1. When you have never loved your parents

There are three main reasons why you are likely to state that you have never loved your parents:

First, your parents may have been 'emotionally unavailable' to you; this means that your emotional needs would not have been satisfied. For example, your parents may have been cold, distant and disinclined to spend much time with you.

Second, there may instead have been *too much* parental involvement with you as a child, such that you always felt overwhelmed and smothered by your parents; this over-involvement prevented you from developing a healthy loving relationship with them. Healthy loving relationships tend to develop where your parents accepted you as a child, but gave you some autonomy and independence so that you could become curious, explore your surroundings, yet still be accepted and protected. If your parents were over-protective and unduly restricted your autonomy, you may have found it difficult to develop a sense of independence. In this case, an unhealthy relationship would tend to develop, because what may pass for 'love' of your parents may simply be the expression of a need to be looked after by them.

Third, it may be that you don't love your parents because you have a very different temperament from them, and perhaps they never accepted you as you are and made allowances for this difference in temperament. In a sense, your parents may have always felt 'foreign' to you.

2. Where you once loved your parents, but have now ceased to love them

This situation occurs because over a long period of time your parents may have failed to meet your deepest desires, and therefore you eventually stopped loving them. You may have some kind of a bond with them, but it's not love. It may be the bond of familiarity, but that isn't love. Love is the strong affectional feelings you have for someone who meets your deepest desires. Love is your emotional response to whatever, or whoever, you value highly.

When you 'fall out of love' with your parents, the main feeling you are likely to experience is guilt, so let's look now at the main reasons why you may feel guilty when you realize that you no longer love your parents.

Reasons why you may feel guilty when you realize that you no longer love your parents

As stated above, you are brought up to believe that you should love your parents, and that there is something wrong with you if you don't. You are given to believe that it is your duty, an obligation, to love your parents; and if you fail to meet your 'obligation' to your parents, you are encouraged to view yourself as something of an uncaring, selfish person. This belief is at the core of your feelings of guilt.

Another reason why you may stop loving your parents is because you feel resentful towards them because of the way they treated you when you were young and in their care. You may put on a façade of lovingness when you and they meet, but you never discuss the reasons for your resentment towards them. The issues don't get discussed, and so you become emotionally distant from them. You seek to avoid your parents because you feel uncomfortable in their presence; any contact you do have with them will be superficial, and consequently you will never get down to having a really open and honest heart-to-heart talk with them to resolve the issues that are bothering you.

If you felt deprived of certain important things when you were in your parents' care, why do you avoid bringing up this issue with them? The answer is that you are afraid you would hurt their feelings if you were to confront them on that issue – for then you would feel guilty about hurting their feelings! So to 'let sleeping dogs lie' becomes your policy. It may seem the easiest way out of avoiding an uncomfortable discussion to let your feelings of resentment and guilt simmer away inside you, but in the long run you will suffer even more if you hang on to these unhealthy emotions.

To summarize, the feeling of guilt can stem from holding either, or both, of the following beliefs:

- 'I absolutely should love my parents, and I am a worthless person if I don't.'

- 'If I were to raise with my parents the issue of why I felt deprived in my childhood of certain things that were important to me, I'd hurt their feelings – and then I'd be a bad person because I'd hurt their feelings.'

The common denominator in virtually all instances of guilt is, as you will see in a moment, a particular form of irrational thinking. Since guilt is the main issue, we will now focus our attention on this.

What exactly is guilt?

At the outset, it is important to distinguish between the *feeling* of guilt, and acknowledging that you *are* guilty of doing something wrong. Generally speaking, a *feeling* of guilt arises from the belief that you have violated ethical, moral or religious codes, which you believe you must not do, and that you are a bad person as a result. A feeling of guilt can also arise when you fail to live up to your principles or hurt other people. In each case, you believe you have done something you must not do and that you are a bad person as a result.

On the other hand, *being* guilty of something simply means accepting responsibility for your actions. Being guilty does not necessarily mean or imply that you must *feel* guilty. The two things – the feeling of guilt, and the fact of having acted wrongly – are quite separate, and you will see in a moment why this is so. You will also see why a feeling of guilt will encourage you to act in ways that are almost invariably self-damaging and counterproductive.

Now, keeping that distinction in mind, you will recall that we introduced you in Chapter 1 to REBT Insight No. 1: You feel as you think. If you apply this Insight to the question of how a feeling of guilt arises, the answer should be clear.

Stated simply, you feel guilty when you believe:

- 'I absolutely should not have done what I did, or should have done what I did not.'

- 'I am a bad person as a consequence.'

These important points should become clearer to you as you study the following example of a problem with guilt. We will introduce you to the problem by way of Key Task No. 1, which we first looked at on pages 8–9.

Key Task No. 1: Getting yourself into a healthy frame of mind emotionally

In this Key Task, we explained why getting yourself into a healthy frame of mind emotionally is a prerequisite for dealing successfully with any kind of emotional problem. The more rational you are in your thinking and behaving, the greater is the likelihood of your managing to cope successfully with the annoyances that inevitably arise when you are dealing with disturbed individuals, including difficult parents. So, now that we know the nature of the problem, let's see how the application of Key Task No. 1 can help you to clarify and resolve the problem of guilt. We have chosen as an example the case of a 20-year-old woman who loved her parents as a child, but now no longer loves them.

'I no longer love my parents!'

Sally was an only child who had been brought up by parents who had married late in life, and who doted on Sally from babyhood until she reached her early teens. Until she reached her teens, Sally recalled that she had always loved her parents because they had been warm, loving and protective towards her for as long as she could remember.

Things began to change for Sally when she was about fourteen years of age. Sally's parents were members of a small and very strict religious sect, and had very definite ideas on how a young teenage girl should behave. Sally had friends of her own age, school friends whom she had grown up with, and who enjoyed a degree of freedom and independence that Sally could only envy. While Sally's friends would meet up and go clothes shopping, or to pop concerts and parties together, Sally's activities were strictly controlled and supervised by her parents. Boyfriends were definitely 'out' as far as Sally was concerned, and she was compelled by her parents to spend more and more time at Bible classes and religious meetings, usually with one or both of her parents present.

By the time Sally came of age, many of her old school friends had largely drifted away as contact between them had become less and less over the years. Consequently, Sally felt lonely and miserable; and she had never fully accepted the religious values her parents and religious leaders had tried to instil into her. She considered that there was something cold and unloving about the way her parents were treating her, and that their outlook was inconsistent with the open warmth and friendliness that Sally had shared and enjoyed with her old school friends, and others she had more recently met outside her narrow family circle. One day, Sally dismayed her parents by announcing that she was leaving home to live in a flat with two friends she had known since her schooldays.

Although Sally was relieved to be free from the restrictive environment of her parents' home, and running her own life, she felt guilty over the fact that she no longer loved her parents. She resented the way they had treated her in her early teens, and the increasingly restrictive regime imposed upon her at a time when most other young adults in her age groups were becoming independent of their parents and choosing their own friends and lifestyles. At the same time, Sally believed that her parents loved her and had acted in what they thought were her best interests. She supposed they meant well, in spite of the obnoxious way they tried to control and restrict her interests, tastes and behaviour. When Sally finally had had enough and left home to share the flat with her friends, she was aware that she no longer loved her parents, and that she felt guilty about that. She felt she had done the right thing for herself in leaving her parents, but why did she have this feeling of guilt over not loving them as she once had?

The A–B–C of Sally's feeling of guilt

(If need be, remind yourself of the A–B–C model of emotional disturbance by looking back at pages 10–11.) If you feel upset at **C** about something that happens at **A**, you will realize by now that **A** does not cause **C**. You know that a **B** exists between **A** and **C**, and that it is this **B** that is at the core of your upset. **B**, you will recall, stands for your Belief System, and consists of the way you view or evaluate what is happening at **A**.

Now Sally has done nothing wrong – after all, she didn't run off with the family silver when she left her parents' home! All that has happened is that she no longer loves her parents, but that is not a crime. So why does Sally feel guilty? She feels guilty because she doesn't love her parents any more – and she thinks she *should*. Let's use the A–B–C model to pinpoint what is going on in Sally's mind:

> **A** stands for the objective fact that Sally no longer loves her parents.
> **B** stands for her beliefs about **A**.
> **C** stands for her feeling of guilt.

What is Sally telling herself at **B** to create her feeling of guilt? From what you know so far, you would expect to find a powerful irrational belief (iB) in the way Sally views her situation. For how else could she feel upset? If Sally merely believed that it was very unfortunate that she no longer loved her parents, she might legitimately feel sorry or disappointed. However, Sally is going beyond feeling sorry, which is the kind of healthy negative feeling that most people would experience if something they had hoped for failed to materialize. Sally feels guilt-ridden and self-deprecating, a very unhealthy negative feeling. So let's see what Sally is telling herself to create this emotionally crippling feeling of guilt.

Sally's iBs

Sally was brought up to believe the commonly held belief that 'you must love your parents', which in Sally's case was strongly reinforced by the religious teachings instilled into her while she was growing up. Thus Sally believes:

- 'I absolutely should love my parents, and because I do not love them as I should, I am a bad person.'

Now, let us remind you of the criteria of irrationality we outlined in

Chapter 1. Irrational beliefs (iBs) consist of absolutist demands or dictates; they are illogical, inconsistent with reality, and lead to poor results emotionally and behaviourally. With these criteria in mind, let's see if Sally would be wise to reconsider her belief that she *should* love her parents.

Disputing Sally's iBs

Let's take the first part of Sally's belief and question it:

1. 'I absolutely *should* love my parents . . .'
(a) *Is this belief logical?* Sally may want to love her parents, but it doesn't logically follow that she absolutely has to. Even if Sally regards it as a moral obligation or injunction to love her parents, she *chooses* that obligation; and, once again, it doesn't logically follow that because one assumes an obligation, that therefore that obligation absolutely must be carried out

(b) *Is this belief consistent with reality?* If this belief was consistent with reality, how could Sally not love her parents? If something must occur, then there would be no way of stopping it! Obviously, there is no law of the universe that commands us to love our parents, for if there were such a law, we'd have no choice but to obey it.

(c) *Will this belief help Sally to achieve her goals?* One of Sally's goals is to achieve a degree of independence from her parents – a goal she has already partly reached. If Sally wishes to retain her independence and to continue deciding for herself how she is going to live her life, she can hardly avoid experiencing a degree of conflict between her goals of personal autonomy and her belief that she absolutely should love her parents. Their values and beliefs tend to point in a different direction from those of Sally, and Sally's parents want her to return to them. It would appear, therefore, that Sally's unqualified demand on herself that she absolutely should love her parents will hinder her in pursuing her personal goals.

Moreover, this belief won't help Sally to discuss her feelings of resentment with her parents and come to some rapprochement with them, with the possibility of eventually rekindling her feelings of love for them.

Now let's examine the second part of Sally's belief about her parents:

2. Sally concludes, '. . . and because I do not love them as I should, I am a bad person.'

(a) *Is this belief logical?* Not at all. How does it logically follow that because Sally doesn't love her parents as she thinks she should, that she becomes a bad person? While it may be bad, meaning unfortunate, if Sally doesn't love her parents, that does not make her a bad person. The conclusion is illogical.

(b) *Is this belief consistent with reality?* Sally's error here is that she identifies her total self with one aspect of her behaviour. That is a gross over-generalization, and not consistent with the facts of reality. In effect, Sally is telling herself, 'I don't love my parents, so that makes me bad. I am nothing more than just an unloving daughter. Nothing else I do or become in the future counts for anything.' Apart from labelling herself a bad person, which is an arbitrary definition anyway, Sally's 'self' is a continually changing, ongoing process that has a past, a present and a future. Her acts, deeds, desires, traits and beliefs are only *aspects* of the total person known as Sally. You may evaluate Sally's traits etc. according to some external standard, but her 'self' is not 'rateable'.

(c) *Will this belief help Sally to achieve her goals?* Sally's goals, or at least some of them, are to maintain her personal autonomy and to decide for herself how to run her life. She may hope, too, that some reconciliation with her parents may one day be possible. However, if she clings to the conviction that she is a bad person because she no longer loves her parents, she is really in a no-win situation. So long as she sticks to her guns and continues to lead a life independent of her parents and refuses to go back to them, she will feel uncomfortable because she sees this as evidence that she no longer loves them, yet believe that she *should* love them. On the other hand, if she were to return to her parents to assuage her feelings of guilt, she might temporarily lessen her severe feelings of worthlessness, but at the cost of sacrificing her independence and autonomy, which she values highly. She would then tend to deprecate herself for that. In any event, Sally is unlikely to feel very loving towards her parents so long as they refuse to accept her right to live her own life as she pleases.

The solution to Sally's dilemma is to challenge her beliefs about herself and her relationship with her parents, see how irrational these beliefs are, and then see what can be done to eliminate them. Once she convinces herself that her belief that she absolutely has to love her parents – and that there must be something fundamentally wrong with her if she doesn't – is untenable, Sally can work hard to correct some of the misconceptions that she has about loving her parents. If Sally also practises challenging and Disputing her iBs, then she will eventually weaken them and replace them with more rational alternative beliefs.

Sally's rational alternative beliefs

Once Sally had convinced herself that loving her parents might be desirable, but that it was hardly a necessity, and that there are no legitimate reasons for her to make herself terribly miserable because she doesn't love them, she could more rationally believe something along the following lines:

- 'I would prefer it if I could go on loving my parents, but I don't have to get what I prefer, and I don't have to love them. Even if I never feel much love for my parents in the future, I am not a worthless person – but instead a fallible human being like everyone else, with my own tastes and values, and who takes responsibility for the right to lead my life as I see fit.'

With these rBs, Sally would feel remorse rather than guilt as a result of the fact that she and her parents could no longer see eye-to-eye over her desire for independence and for the freedom to make her own decisions in life; and she would feel sorry, rather than terribly upset, over the fact that she no longer found her parents very lovable. Instead of seeing herself as a totally bad person for not loving her parents, Sally would now take the view that she can accept herself as a fallible human being who doesn't always, or even mainly, have to be right in everything she does in order to consider herself worthy of happiness.

As a result of giving up her guilt-creating beliefs, Sally would open up the possibility of getting along better with her parents than before. Once she had freed herself from their influence on what she should think and how she should behave and no longer saw herself as a rebel against her parents' ideas and the kind of life they had insisted that she lead, Sally could make a start on constructing a healthier relationship with her parents, and look forward to living her own life in a more enjoyable manner.

At this point, let us see what has been achieved. If your experience parallels that of Sally, and you feel guilty over the knowledge that you no longer love your parents, we hope that you will find our treatment of the question of guilt both illuminating and helpful. So long as you retain the belief that you absolutely should love your parents, and you feel guilty or self-hating because you don't love them, you are unlikely to acquire the frame of mind that will possibly help you to achieve a rapprochement with them. Acceptance and understanding of both yourself and others, especially your close relatives, is a prerequisite for finding a way to get along with them. Overcoming unhealthy negative feelings, and replacing them with more rational, healthy attitudes, helps pave the way towards enabling you to cope with your difficult parents in a less stressful manner.

If guilt feelings have been a problem for you, we suggest that before you continue with the next sections, you satisfy yourself that you fully understand how you create your feelings of guilt, and accept that you need never denigrate yourself because of them.

Let's return now to the case of Sally. She has abandoned her earlier iBs that she absolutely should love her parents, and has overcome her unhealthy feelings of guilt over the knowledge that she no longer loves them. Using the example we gave you in Chapter 1 of how Gary overcame his resentment of the way his father treated him, Sally could tackle her own resentment of the way her parents had treated her. Both guilt and resentment are unhealthy negative emotions. So long as they are present, they won't help you to improve your relationship with your parents. So if either (or both) of these problems are currently troubling you, we suggest that you tackle them using the Disputing methods we have shown you in this and the previous chapter, before moving on to the next sections where we discuss Key Tasks No. 2 and No. 3. When you are dealing with difficult parents, it's important that you carry out your Three Key Tasks in the order in which they are presented. Understanding you parents and aiming to get on better with them is your objective; that also is Sally's objective. So far, Sally has accomplished Key Task No. 1. She has acquired the right frame of mind to enable her to deal with her parents in a constructive manner. However, she still has some work to do before she gets within sight of her ultimate goal. So, if you are now ready to proceed with us to the next stage, let's see how Sally would go about accomplishing Key Tasks No. 2 and No. 3.

Key Task No. 2: *Understanding and accepting your parents with their difficult traits and behaviour*

Understanding your parents involves trying to see the world through their eyes. How do your parents think and feel about you now? How did they think and feel about you as they brought you up?

You will recall that we began this chapter by distinguishing two different kinds of parental upbringing. On the one hand, you may have had the kind of parents who were under-involved with you in the sense of not showing you much love. They may have been cold and distant because they did not have loving parents themselves, and therefore found it difficult to show love because they really hadn't had much love shown to them as children, or had a good model of loving parents to emulate. It's easy to condemn your parents for not being as loving as you would have wished. However, if you had been brought up as they were by their parents, would you have done any better? Once you put yourself in your parents' shoes and imagine how you would have come to view the world given the kind of upbringing they experienced, you may find it easier to feel sorry for them, rather than blame them, for being unable to show their feelings. It isn't so long ago that some people were taught to view displays of emotion towards their children and grandchildren as weaknesses. Little wonder, then, that they felt uncomfortable about showing their emotions and decided to avoid the discomfort of doing so.

No doubt you can easily see the irrationality of believing that it is a sign of weakness to display certain emotions such as showing love to one's children or grandchildren, and that one must avoid such weaknesses. However, your present task is not to Dispute your parents' iBs but to understand and to make allowances for the fact that your parents were frequently the victims of iBs that they were taught during their young and impressionable years, and that they were largely powerless to resist.

On the other hand, you may have had parents like Sally's who were over-involved, and who unduly restricted you as you sought to acquire a degree of autonomy and independence. Such parents feel anxious about their ability to cope in what they see as a hostile world, and consequently become over-protective. They are intolerant of children's individuality because they fear that 'terrible' things will happen to them if they start to think for themselves, acquire 'dangerous' views, and stray from the controlled and narrow way of life they have mapped out for you to follow.

Sally's parents strongly held iBs such as, 'The world is a wicked and sinful place and people absolutely should behave better than they do; and since they do not, they are awful and horrible; and since we can't stand the thought of Sally being affected by such wickedness, we must protect her from it, or terrible things will happen to her if we fail.' Sally wanted to Dispute he parents' iBs; but wisely, she resisted the temptation! She was shown that she would achieve better results at this stage by conveying to her parents that she understood why they held the beliefs they did, and that while she didn't enjoy the restrictions imposed upon her, she didn't condemn them in any way for what they did, or failed to do, as a result of the beliefs they held at the time.

The important point here is that Sally realized that people respond to what is going on in their own heads, and therefore that demanding that her parents be different would be counterproductive. If you *demand* that your parents be different, or change their ways because you don't like the way they are, you are behaving irrationally yourself. You may legitimately prefer that your parents had behaved differently in the past, you may even hope that they will change in the future, but if you demand that they change their ways because you think they 'should', then you are acting irrationally – because you will make yourself angry when they fail to behave as you demand that they 'should'. You will also sabotage your chances of establishing a better relationship with them. Understanding your parents doesn't just mean understanding how they came to be the way they are; it also implies accepting them as they are.

The key point here is that you can accept, not condemn, your difficult parents while not accepting certain *aspects* of their behaviour. Sally, for example, didn't like the way her parents were over-protective of her and restricted her personal freedom to the point where she had virtually no independence. She not only didn't like the way her parents treated her; she resented it. She then felt guilty over the fact that she no longer loved her parents. However, once she was able to overcome her feelings of guilt and to give up her resentment, Sally was able to take her first steps to understanding and accepting her parents.

To begin with, Sally learned that a human being is an incredibly complex process with innumerable acts, traits and purposes that change over time. Some of your acts are good, some are bad; and some are neither. Sally thought this over and agreed that there are no totally 'good' or 'bad' people. Then she concluded, 'That means that my parents are not totally ''good'' or ''bad'' people because of what they did and didn't do over their lifetime. They're just people who at times acted well, but who at other times acted less well than they might. But then, don't we all?'

If you put somebody down for not living up to your expectations, anger or resentment results. When you put yourself down as a total person, guilt and/or depression follow. Can you see now that it makes no sense to identify a person with his/her behaviour and that you can accept the person without accepting that person's behaviour? It makes good sense to accept other people unconditionally, and that goes especially for your difficult parents! That doesn't mean that you necessarily like them, or agree with them. It simply means that you accept your parents as fallible people, with the right to live and run their own lives as they choose.

You can help to strengthen this more rational attitude by conveying to your parents in various ways that you fully accept them. For example, you can deliberately act lovingly towards them rather than angrily when they complain about or criticize your lifestyle. You can train yourself to talk to them in a manner that conveys warmth and understanding of their point of view and feelings, without necessarily agreeing with them. This does not guarantee that your relationship with your parents will become, as they say, 'lovey-dovey', but your non-blaming, accepting attitude towards your parents may eventually rub off on them and encourage them to respond positively to your constructive attempts to build a closer or warmer relationship.

To round off this section, we would stress the very important and logical point that fully accepting others implies that you fully accept yourself as well. If you don't accept yourself, you can hardly expect to make a success of accepting other people, especially those who are close to you, such as your parents.

When you unconditionally accept yourself, you choose to acknowledge fully that you have the right to live and to make yourself as happy as you can whether or not you do well, act competently, receive love from somebody, or have some admirable or outstanding quality. You simply choose to accept yourself, with no 'ifs' or 'buts'.

Once you see that it makes good sense to accept yourself totally, with your flaws and failings, you will see that it makes equally good sense to accept other people and their failings. That doesn't mean that you necessarily like them, or agree with them. As we have already pointed out, you can accept people without accepting certain behaviour. You simply accept yourself and others as fallible humans with the right to live and to run their own lives as they choose.

Key Task No. 3: Acting in an enlightened self-interested way towards your parents

In Chapter 1 we explained what acting in a self-interested way really means. In Key Task No. 3, you will bring together the insights you have acquired as you worked through Key Tasks No. 1 and No. 2, and apply these to the present task of acting in an enlightened self-interested way towards your parents, with the aim of getting along better with them.

In Key Task No. 1, you worked to eliminate the iBs that impeded you from dealing in a rational manner with the knowledge that you don't love your parents. Then in Key Task No. 2, you learned what it means to understand and accept your parents. How you decide to treat them from now on will depend upon the response you get from them. Once more, we will take the case of Sally to illustrate a number of important points.

How Sally communicated with her parents

Truly understanding and accepting your parents and their shortcomings means that, regardless of what kind of parents they are, and irrespective of the kind of upbringing you had, you fully respect their right to be the way they are. Once you clearly convey that you fully accept them, you can then discuss in a non-blaming manner the issues that come between you.

Let's see how Sally began her attempt to improve relations with her parents. Up until then, Sally and her parents had been on speaking terms, but there had been hardly any real communication between them, and a number of important issues needed to be discussed before any improvement in their relationship was likely to materialize.

Sally initiated the process of getting back on better terms with her parents by inviting them to tea at her flat, and her invitation was accepted. Her parents had not previously visited Sally in her own home, and Sally wanted them to see for themselves that she was managing her life in a sensible manner and looking after herself.

In what turned out to be an extended conversation, Sally explained why she had decided to leave her parents' home and live on her own. Using what she had learned as she worked through Key Tasks No. 1 and No. 2, Sally conveyed to her parents that she fully understood their concern when she moved out of their home and into a flat, and the anxiety they experienced over the 'terrible' things they were sure would happen to her. Without deriding her parents' beliefs in any way, Sally explained why she felt unable to accept them. She explained to her parents why she felt they had been too loving, too concerned about her welfare, and as a consequence had restricted her life in ways that tended to inhibit her from developing as an individual. Sally gently explained to them that they had been too over-protective towards her, and that for her own sake she decided she had to get out.

Sally made it clear to her parents that when she moved out of their home, she was not rejecting them, but instead asserting her right to direct her own life as a responsible adult in a manner consistent with her goals and aspirations. She especially emphasized that she didn't doubt for a single moment that her parents loved her, and that she believed they had always acted in what they thought were her best interests.

Through having this frank and open discussion with her parents of those issues that had not previously been resolved, Sally said that she hoped that all three of them might now reach a better mutual understanding. Sally assured her parents that she cared about them, and that she looked forward to exchanging visits with them, on a regular basis.

The outcome was that Sally achieved her objective. After some initial hesitation, Sally's parents saw that what Sally had done made sense from her point of view. Moreover, they found Sally's caring attitude towards them reassuring, and they agreed to meet on a regular basis. They told Sally that while they still would have preferred her to move back in with them, they realized that Sally had her reasons for wanting to live on her own, and they accepted her decision. They were happy to know that Sally cared about them and were delighted that she wished to have regular contact with them in the future. Sally's father was very pleased to accept Sally's offer of occasional help in her parents' garden, an activity that he and Sally used to enjoy sharing when Sally lived with her parents. For her part, Sally's mother welcomed Sally's suggestion that she accompany her mother whenever she went clothes shopping, because, as her mother remarked, 'I liked having Sally with me when I went to buy clothes for myself. She always did have good taste when it came to clothes, and she knew a bargain when she saw one.'

Communicating with your parents

Several key points may be extracted from Sally's efforts to get on better terms with her parents, but not all attempts to improve relations with your difficult parents will result in outcomes as happy as Sally's. Some parents, for a variety of reasons, will be adamantly against having any contact at all with their adult offspring; and with some adult offspring, the feeling will be reciprocated. In these circumstances, you may have to be content with a fairly low-key relationship with your parents, or even none at all.

However, if there is some desire for a better relationship and a degree of willingness on both sides to take steps to achieve it, quite satisfactory outcomes are possible. If you consider there is a reasonable chance of restoring a relationship that you once had with your parents, you may find it helpful to bear these and the following points in mind.

If you are aiming to restore communication with your parents, it is not generally advisable to criticize them for expressing views or opinions with which you disagree. Instead, try to see what they are saying from their frame of reference and convey that you understand them. Try to understand the feelings behind their words. Reflect back to them what you understand they mean – for example, 'Am I right in thinking that you thought I was being inconsiderate and selfish when I went on holiday the day you entered hospital?' That is what 'empathic understanding' means – in other words, it aims to help each person in an argument or discussion to appreciate the meaning behind the other person's words. Until each person knows what the other means, a fruitful dialogue is unlikely to ensue. If the differences between you appear to stem from different expectations about how parents and their adult offspring should behave, try to empathize with your parents by imagining how you would have seen the world if you had shared the same background and values, and had the same upbringing as they had. If your parents see that you are not denying the validity of their feelings and experiences, and that you really do understand and appreciate their point of view, they will be less motivated to impose it on you. When your parents feel they have been heard and that you understand what they have lived through and learned throughout their lifetime, the way may then be open for you to explain calmly why you hold a different point of view. It isn't a question of proving who is 'right' or who is 'wrong' – such an adversarial stance will get you nowhere. If your parents accuse you and condemn you for your misdeeds or shortcomings, don't react in kind! If they damn you and put you down for your failings, they do so for basically the same reasons as you yourself might have were it not for your more rational attitude.

Show your parents that you understand how they feel, and even indicate that if you saw yourself as they see you, you could even agree with them: 'If I were in your shoes, I'd criticize me too!' Make allowances for the way your parents perceive you and your errors, and strive to accept them as you would like them to accept you.

We are not advocating that you simply lie down and let your parents walk all over you. You can stand up for yourself when your parents address you in a hostile, disparaging or manipulative way without

41

getting dragged into their 'game'. Politely offer to agree to differ, and don't allow yourself to be pulled into a shouting match.

If you cultivate empathic listening, each of you can come to appreciate how the other is right from their own perspective, and there is then a better chance that your parents will see your point of view as well as their own.

However, if your best efforts are to no avail, and your parents persist in trying to prove how right they are and how wrong you are, the worst thing you can do is to get angry with them. As you will recall from the example in Chapter 1 in which Gary got angry over the way his father continually criticized him, anger begets anger and tends to drive people farther apart. Besides, simmering anger can have unfortunate consequences for your physical health. If your parents fail to respond positively to your attempts to resolve the differences between you, and continue to argue with you and refuse to accept your right to your views, you don't have to feel angry. The rational alternative to anger is annoyance. If you are frustrated in your efforts to improve communication with your parents, it's healthy to feel displeased or annoyed as well as sorry when this happens. Don't think that you should be calm or obliged to turn the other cheek; be firm but fair.

'You've hurt my feelings!'

Based on your understanding of REBT, you will readily see that people's words or attitudes cannot hurt you or humiliate you unless you allow them to. If your parents accuse you of hurting their feelings, how should you respond? Generally speaking, we consider it inadvisable to launch into a lecture at this point on REBT Insight no. 1! If your parents are into middle age or beyond, they are unlikely to appreciate your attempt to lecture them – and still less to understand it. They are more likely to see your attempt at explanation as a ploy to deny the validity of their feelings or an attempt to play down their significance. So, spare them your analysis and instead acknowledge that they feel hurt, and express your regret without concurring with their view that you caused their 'hurt' feelings. If your parents are fairly young in their outlook and reasonably well educated, you may see an opportunity to venture an explanation of how 'hurt' feelings arise – if not, keep silent!

Your best bet is to keep your cool and try to be empathic with your parents when they are being difficult and frustrating you. It's irrational to expect them to be different from the way they actually are; accept them with their failings.

Acting in your own best interests

If your parents react positively and show some understanding and acceptance of your views, they may convey signs of wanting to establish closer emotional ties with you. If so, well and good. This may involve you in spending more time with them, helping them out in various ways, and so on. It will then be up to you to decide how much of your own time you are willing to devote to your parents. If it appears to you that some measure of self-sacrifice is called for or implied, you may need to weigh up the pros and cons of spending time with your parents as against devoting that time to pursuing your own interests and projects. Some kind of mutually agreed compromise may be in both your best interests, but whatever arrangement is agreed can always be changed or renegotiated in the light of changing circumstances.

Enlightened self-interest, as we pointed out in Chapter 1, is a fine trait for both you and your parents to aim for, but when self-interest is displaced and replaced by self-centredness on the part of either or both of you, beware! Self-centredness goes beyond believing that not only has one a right to be happy, to that the world owes one a living, and that other people have an obligation to be of service – regardless of their own wishes in the matter. Should this attitude be held by your parents, you may find it necessary to distance yourself emotionally from them, but at the same time to refrain from condemning them. Don't sever all contact with your parents; instead, make it clear to them that while you recognize their legitimate rights and interests, you will give priority to standing up for your own rights and following your own interests until such time as they are prepared to acknowledge your legitimate claims to put your own interests on a par with theirs.

Generally, it is more advantageous for both you and your parents to be on reasonably amicable terms with each other rather than at loggerheads. At the very least, it will be less stressful. However, you don't have to feel particularly amicable or loving towards them to be able to get on with them, nor do you have to feel guilty if you don't love them. A common willingness to acknowledge one another's right to live and let live without an undue amount of mutual complaint or criticism will go a long way towards enabling you to create and maintain a reasonably workable relationship with them.

In Chapter 3, we look at the opposite side of the coin, for here we examine the situation where you love your parents 'too much'. We explain what is meant by loving 'too much', and show you how to deal with the problems that frequently arise when that happens.

3

How to Love Your Parents
without Loving Them 'Too Much'

We had better explain at the outset what we mean by loving 'too much'. You might even question whether it is possible to love, or be loved, 'too much'. After all, throughout history, love has inspired poetry, drama, literature, and practically every kind of music. In operatic arias, love has been the inspiration behind both tragedies and comedies. Newspapers and magazines devote many column inches to advising their perplexed readers how to recognize love, how to get it, and how to hold on to it once they have found it. Entire pages in local newspapers are filled with personal ads from people looking for love; and agony aunts are kept busy advising the lovelorn and the broken-hearted how to cope with the loss of love and how to win it back.

So highly valued is love in our society that it has come to be regarded by many as a cure for practically everything that ails them. So in the face of this apparently overwhelming desire or need for love, how can anyone seriously imagine that loving 'too much' can ever be a problem?

Well, strange as it may seem, you *can* love and be loved too much. However, as you will see presently, it isn't so much real love itself that creates problems between you and your parents when you love them 'too much' or the other way round; rather, it is the unhealthy form that the love between you takes that damages your relationship.

In what follows, we consider two basic situations that illustrate what we mean by loving 'too much'. We will show you what happens to the quality of your relationship with your parents when you love them too much; then we will show you why it happens. Loving your parents too much doesn't come about by accident. Unhealthy patterns of relating to your parents in your adult life, such as over-involvement and dependency, stem from attitudes you acquired towards your parents that originated in your childhood. As a child you were dependent upon your parents for survival; you needed them to look after you and protect you. While these attitudes of dependency may have been appropriate and healthy when you were a child, they begin to appear more and more unrealistic and self-defeating once you've left your childhood behind you.

44

If irrational views dominate your thinking, and continue to dominate it throughout your adult life, the outcome in terms of how you and your parents interact becomes almost predictable. A major part of this chapter will focus on showing you how to identify your early acquired iBs, and how you can eliminate and replace them with a more rational outlook that will help you and your parents to move towards a healthier, more mature type of loving relationship.

Let's briefly look now at the two basic situations we mentioned a moment ago that illustrate what happens when you love your parents 'too much'.

Loving 'too much'

1. You believe you are dependent upon your parents

In this situation, you love your parents too much because you are over-dependent upon them for their love or approval. You see yourself as too weak an individual to make your own decisions, to cope with life on your own, and so you allow them to take over. You rely on them, and as a result you don't acquire the coping skills to enable you to look after yourself. You continually go to them for help and advice, and they continually help you out, mainly because of their own feelings of guilt, but also because of their own need to be needed.

It is your dependency upon them – your need for their love and approval, together with their dire need to be needed – rather than loving 'too much' that harms your relationship with your parents and diminishes the quality of life for both you and them. Even if you are physically handicapped to some degree, and require assistance at times, you don't have to feel dependent upon your parents for everything. There are still things you can do for yourself. If you have a healthy attitude, you will find it personally beneficial to do as much as you can for yourself and to be as independent of others as you can within the limits of your physical capacity.

However, your belief that you can't lead a more independent existence doesn't necessarily come from some kind of physical impairment, but instead from an over-protective childhood that you have allowed to continue into adult life – and that you now sustain because you still cling to the iB that you need your parents' approval and support to manage your life.

One unfortunate consequence is that if you get married, your marriage becomes 'triangulated'; in other words, you fail to achieve an adult relationship with your partner because your parents become over-involved as well. The marriage, then, isn't just between you and your partner; it's between you, your partner and your parents – a triangular relationship. The chances of your partner tolerating that situation for long are slim, and the marriage is quite likely to end with your partner leaving it.

Now, let's look at the second situation.

2. *Your parents believe they are dependent upon you*

In this case, it is your parents who are weak; they either can't, or won't, be independent. They make out that they need you to look after them, even though they may be in perfectly good health. Perhaps they have convinced you that you owe it to them to look after them. At any rate, you believe that you *have to* help them – after all, they are you parents. It's now you who has this need to be needed. Your rush round to them for the slightest thing. They need shopping, so you get their shopping. Or they have a headache and don't feel very well; so you rush round and commiserate with them. You end up by being at their beck and call. If you fail to heed their demands for help, you become a bad person in your own eyes. Looking after your parents' every need becomes your vocation in life.

If you compare these two situations, you will see that in the first situation your parents are always bailing you out of trouble, taking decisions for you and so on, whereas in the second situation you bail them out of trouble. In other words, your roles are reversed. In both situations, the relationship is an unhealthy one: in the first one, they 'baby' you; in the second, you 'baby' them. Unable to distinguish being needed from being loved, you live with the fear of not being needed by your parents some day in the future. So you press on, lavishing all your time and attention on them in the hope that nothing will happen to change your obsession that your parents need you.

When the situation is the other way round and you are the dependent one in the relationship, your parents continue to put themselves out for you because of their neurotic need to be needed. They may also feel guilty at having brought you into a harsh world that they believe was always going to be too difficult for you to learn to cope with, and so they try to make it up to you by looking after you and discouraging you from becoming independent of them for as long as they can.

If you are in this situation and believe that you need someone stronger than yourself on whom to rely, and are happy to have your parents take on that responsibility, so be it. However, you would do well to remember that if you depend on others, you never know when they will cease being dependable. Your parents being older than you will probably die before you will, or they may become incapacitated and totally unable to look after themselves, let alone you. What will you do then? Dependency leads to less and less confidence in your ability to look after yourself, and invariably leaves you to a considerable degree at the mercy of others and external events over which you have no control. Is that what you really want?

You may have been over-protected as a child, but you are no longer a child. Are you prepared to give up your individuality and the many things *you* want to do and could do with the one life you definitely have? Ask yourself: is being dependent on my parents what I truly want for myself? If it isn't, you don't have to remain in this position. There are millions of people out there in the world, and many possibilities for living a more enjoyable life for yourself once you break free from that ever-narrowing circle of total dependency on others that you have created for yourself.

If you want to free yourself from a life of dependency on your parents and to become an autonomous adult able to relate to your parents in healthier way, you can. However, it will require you to work at it – you can't break the habits of a lifetime overnight – but the eventual reward will be worth the effort. Let's see what we can do to help you to escape from this suffocating dependency, and at the same time help your parents to abandon their self-sacrificing martyrdom. Excessive self-sacrifice rarely does anyone much good, regardless of who is doing the sacrificing. If your situation is a type 1 scenario where you are dependent upon your parents, you will learn how to love your parents from a position of strength, not weakness. If it's a type 2 scenario in which you 'baby' your parents, your goal is to continue to care *about* them, not to take care *of* them.

Dependent and co-dependent

If you are psychologically dependent upon your parents in the sense of allowing them to take responsibility for running your life, they become co-dependants, psychologically speaking. A co-dependant is someone who has developed an unhealthy pattern of relating to a dependent person. Generally, the behaviour of the co-dependant reinforces the behaviour of the dependent individual, with the result that he or she becomes even more dependent upon the co-dependant. The dependent individual has a need to be looked after, while the co-dependant has a need to be needed. As a result, both their 'needs' mesh together; the one need feeds the other. You will appreciate, therefore, that if you are the dependent person in the situation and you begin to move away from your habitual ways of behaving towards your co-dependent parents, they will tend to see this as upsetting a pattern to which they have become accustomed – and in consequence are likely to become anxious over the possibility of not being needed by you in the future. It is advisable for you to be aware of that possibility. Later on, we will show you how to understand your parents' role in this situation and how you can encourage them to encourage *you* to stand on your own two feet. At first, though, your parents may well experience the pain of rejection as you struggle to break free; they may well feel that you no longer love them. Your task won't be made any easier by the knowledge that 'suffering for love' is romanticized by our culture! Immature relationships of all kinds are constantly glorified and glamorized by the media in our society with hardly any let up. This means that if you try to break out of your unhealthy pattern of relating to your parents, you may encounter resistance.

Let's focus our attention now on the kind of beliefs that you acquired in the past and that now keep you in a state of dependency upon your parents. This hasn't happened because they conditioned you when you were a child to hold these beliefs, although that may well be how you originally acquired them. When you were a child, it was natural for you to be dependent upon your parents; you needed them then to look after you. But today, as an adult, you don't need your parents – you only think you do. You choose to allow yourself to be over-dependent upon them rather than taking control of your own life because you still cling to your early acquired beliefs that you are a dependent individual who needs someone to look after you or take decisions for you. Probably your parents over-protected you when you were a child in their care, and for their own reasons they chose to continue to look after you in your 'best interests' (or so they believed) long after there was any realistic need for them to do so. They are therefore unlikely to encourage you to become less dependent upon them.

So, what are you and your parents telling yourselves to maintain this unhealthy situation? The iBs that follow are typical of those we find among over-dependent people and the co-dependants who minister to them.

The iBs of over-dependent people

Overly dependent individuals maintain their dependent status by strongly believing:

- 'I absolutely must continue to rely and depend on other people. Because I remain weak in this respect, I shall continue to need and to rely on significant others to enable me to survive in this stressful and difficult world.'

The iBs of co-dependent people

Co-dependants maintain their co-dependent status by strongly believing:

- 'I can rate myself as a good and worthy person only if I unstintingly devote myself to the welfare of significant others, and always put their needs and interests above my own, because that is the only way I can get people generally to approve of me.'

Can you see that so long as you and your parents hold to these iBs (or close variants of them), there is little chance of either of you being able to break the pattern of dependency that has become the established way in which you relate to each other, even if you want to change it?

Do you recall REBT Insight No. 1 that we introduced on page 10? It stated that you feel as you think, and that thinking, feeling and behaving are all interrelated. It follows that if you want to change the way you and your parents have habitually related to each other, you need to change the way you think about your relationship. That is the first step; once that is accomplished, your next steps consist in working at changing the ways you interact with your parents in order to establish new, healthier ways of relating to them. First, though, you need to challenge and Dispute the beliefs you presently hold.

We shall illustrate the procedure by means of the following example. As in previous chapters, we shall structure our discussion around the Three Key Tasks.

An example of over-dependency on parental approval in a young adult

Peter was an only child of well-off parents who had always been over-protective of him from the time he was born. He was by no means physically weak, and he certainly did not need the extra attention his parents insisted on lavishing upon him.

By the time Peter was 20, he had a good job with a computer company and felt ready to leave home. He decided that he was competent enough to look after himself and that it was time he went to live on his own and to stand on his own two feet. Peter loved his parents and appreciated what they had done for him, but he felt restricted by their over-attentiveness and over-concern, and he wanted to experience life more fully than he could within the confining atmosphere of his parents' home.

Yet Peter was afraid that if he left home there was no way he could do that without appearing ungrateful to his parents for all that they had done for him. Peter knew his parents well enough to know that they would feel terribly hurt if he told them of his desire to leave home and become independent. And if he did anything to hurt his parents, what would that say about him? Peter couldn't stand the thought of incurring his parents' disapproval.

The result was that Peter kept putting off what he called the 'evil day' when he would be obliged to tell his parents of his decision to leave them. Peter definitely wanted to leave his parents and become independent, but he also felt that he must have their approval first; he also knew that if he left home, his parents would take it badly. Peter hated the thought that his parents would think he didn't love them any more. That was what Peter felt most upset about, because he would feel terribly ashamed if he was seen as the cause of his parents' distress. Unaware of how he was putting himself into a no-win situation, Peter felt at a complete loss to know how to resolve his dilemma.

Peter's iBs

Peter was shown that his dilemma stemmed from the way in which he viewed the situation. Peter's reluctance to go for what he wanted sprang from a variant of what we term 'Major Irrational Belief No. 1'. There are three Major Irrational Beliefs. You haven't met them yet, so we will now highlight Major Irrational Belief No. 1, and then discuss the particular variant of it that was at the root of Peter's shame and anxiety.

Major Irrational Belief No. 1

'Because it would be highly preferable if I were outstandingly competent and/or loved, I absolutely should and must be that. It's awful when I am not, and therefore I am a worthless individual.'

Peter's variant of this is essentially:

- 'I absolutely must have my parents' approval – or at least avoid their active disapproval. If I fail, they would think badly of me – and that would mean I'm no good.'

If you believe that you absolutely must win the approval of people who are important to you, then you are going to be in a state of perpetual anxiety as you dwell on the ever-present possibility that one day you won't do well. How will you then feel when those people, whose approval you believe you must have, make it clear that they strongly disapprove of you? The answer is, you will feel ashamed. Why? Because you agree with their evaluation of you! You put yourself down. If you didn't, you wouldn't feel ashamed.

Both anxiety and shame are unhealthy because not only do they spring from iBs but also because neither are likely to help you attain your goals in life. Apart from that, these negative emotions are uncomfortable and unnecessary. So, how do you change them? You should know by now that you can change an emotion by modifying the thinking processes that created it. So, let's look at Peter's belief that he has to have his parents' approval. Can this belief be supported? Let's look at it in the context of Key Task No. 1.

Key Task No. 1: Getting yourself into a healthy frame of mind emotionally

The core of Peter's problem lay in his demand that he must not lose his parents' approval. This was what he really meant when he told himself, 'I must not hurt my parents.' This led him to feel anxious at the prospect of leaving home, for if they withdrew their approval of him for leaving home and if they felt he had hurt them by doing so – as he knew they would – he would feel ashamed of himself. For Peter, to hurt those he loved was unforgivable.

If Peter could overcome his shame, he would then be in a much

51

better position to re-evaluate his belief that he must have his parents' approval, and therefore avoid risking their disapproval for anything he did in the future that might clash with their ideas or feelings.

Now suppose for a moment that you have a problem similar to Peter's. A good question to ask yourself is, 'What different feelings would I like to experience and what different actions would I like to take, if someone I love disapproves of me for something I have done, and I feel ashamed as a result?' Why is this an important question to ask yourself? The answer is that your goal, rationally speaking, should be to reach the point where you can do what you think is right for you and to risk displeasing someone you love – not just your parents – without feeling in any way ashamed of yourself. If you merely manage to avoid feeling ashamed when you displease your parents, but you still draw back from risking the disapproval of your lover, your partner, or other significant people in your life when you wish to make some change that is important to you, then you haven't really overcome the basic problem – namely, how to refuse to be ashamed about your choices.

Let's see now how the application of Key Task No. 1 helped Peter to set about answering that question. In Chapter 1, we outlined the criteria you can use to determine whether a given belief is irrational or not; remind yourself of these criteria by looking back at pages 15–16.

Disputing Peter's iBs

Let's look again at Peter's iBs concerning his need for his parents' approval:

- 'I absolutely must have my parents' approval – or at least avoid their active disapproval. If I fail, they would think badly of me – and that would mean I'm no good.'

(a) *Is this belief logical?* The first part clearly isn't. Even if Peter strongly wants his parents' approval and wishes to avoid their disapproval, it doesn't logically follow that he absolutely must get what he wants. Nor does it logically follow that if he fails to achieve what he wants, and his parents think badly of him, that he is worthless.

(b) *Is this belief consistent with reality?* No. Because if there were some universal law that Peter absolutely had to have his parents' approval at all times, then he would; he would have no option but to have their approval! Clearly, he does have the option because he knows he can lose their approval, and is afraid of losing it. So this belief is not realistic; it does not correspond with the facts of the situation.

Furthermore, as we have pointed out in several previous examples of Disputing, you cannot legitimately label anyone as 'good', 'bad' or 'worthless' on the basis of possessing some trait that other people deem 'good', 'bad' or 'worthless'.

(c) *Will this belief help Peter to achieve his goals?* If one of Peter's goals is to gain his parents' approval for every decision he makes in life regardless of his own preferences, then this belief will do nicely! However, we know that Peter wishes to break free from his over-dependence upon his parents' approval, so this belief will not help him to achieve his goals.

Peter's rational alternative beliefs

If Peter works hard at vigorously Disputing his iB that he must have his parents' approval before acting on his own behalf, and that it is shameful if he incurs their disapproval, he will weaken his iB and eventually cease to believe it. Of course, this will take lots of hard work and practice.

For the moment, though, let's see what rational alternative beliefs Peter acquired as a result of his Disputing efforts outlined above:

- 'I would certainly prefer to have my parents' approval for decisions that are important to me, but I don't absolutely have to have it. If my parents think badly of me, that is unfortunate and regrettable, but there is no reason why they must not think badly of me. They are entitled to their views, as I am to mine. I don't have to accept their evaluation of my actions, and I am certainly not a bad person. I am a fallible human being who, over the course of my lifetime, will perform many actions, some of which may be rated good, some bad, and some neutral. However, my totality, my "essence", is "un-rateable".'

Provided Peter truly believes these more rational formulations and sticks to them, he will experience regret rather than shame when his parents (or other significant people) openly express disapproval of him. He may still *prefer* to have his parents' approval, but because he no longer attaches his personal worth to getting it, he will no longer feel anxious at the prospect of losing it.

When you are the co-dependant

Now, let's look briefly at the other way in which you can 'love' your parents 'too much'. Here, the roles are reversed; this time, your parents are in the over-dependent role. They believe that they are unable to take their own decisions, and need you to look after them. If you hold to the idea that you *have* to put your parents' interests first, that it should be your vocation in life, then you beome the obliging co-dependent person in the relationship. Since many adult offspring today are faced with precisely this problem with their parents, it is necessary to discuss this issue.

So, let's apply the criteria of rationality with which you are now familiar to the beliefs typically held by co-dependants.

The iBs of co-dependent people

In their most general form, they can be stated as follows:

- 'I can rate myself as a good and worthy person only if I unstintingly devote myself to the welfare of significant others, and always put their needs and interests above my own, because that is the only way I can get people generally to approve of me.'

We can shorten and rephrase the iB to highlight the essential points that apply in the case of someone who has become a co-dependant to over-dependent parents, thus:

- 'I absolutely must devote myself unstintingly to the welfare of my parents. If I fail, they won't approve of me, and therefore I would be a bad person.'

Compare that with Peter's iB that he must have his parents' approval:

- 'I absolutely must have my parents' approval – or at least avoid their active disapproval. If I fail, they would think badly of me – and that would mean I'm no good.'

The iBs are virtually the same, except in the feelings that result from them. In the second statement given here, Peter's iBs will probably lead him to feel shame when he fails to win his parents' approval or incurs their disapproval. The first statement – the iB that you must unstintingly devote yourself to your parents' welfare – may lead to

54

feelings of guilt when you don't do what you demand of yourself that you must do. Notice how shame and guilt stem from the same type of thinking. Both involve doing something considered bad, stupid or wrong. The difference is this: shame comes from receiving the disapproval of others; guilt comes from receiving one's own disapproval. However, the conclusion is identical in both cases: 'I'm no good'.

Since we have already shown you how to Dispute Peter's iB that he must have his parents' approval or otherwise he is a bad person, you could try out your own Disputing skills now by tackling the iB that you must devote yourself to your parents' welfare – and that if you don't, you are no good. Then, having done that, what rational alternative beliefs could you adopt about your relationship with your parents? We suggest the following ones.

Rational alternative beliefs to the iB that you absolutely must devote yourself unstintingly to serving your parents' interests

- 'While I may choose to devote myself to my parents' interests, at least for a time, there is no reason why I absolutely must do so. Moreover, I can review the situation periodically and make whatever changes I consider to be in my own best interests, while taking due account of their interests. In any case, whether or not I devote myself to my parents' welfare, and regardless of whether I succeed or fail to gain their approval for my actions, I am never a bad person. I am me, a fallible human with innumerable traits and characteristics that change over time. I may at times do well and make wise decisions, and at other times I may do badly and make poor decisions. In any event, while my actions may be rated according to some standard, I – my personhood or totality – can never be rated or measured in any way whatsoever.'

Instead of experiencing a feeling of guilt when your parents express their disapproval of your attempts to attend devotedly to their welfare, you will experience *remorse* if you infer that in fact you failed to put your best efforts into looking after their welfare as you had intended. The reason that you feel remorse rather than guilt is because your belief about the situation is now rational: in effect, you believe, 'I don't like failing to live up to my standards to devote myself as wholeheartedly to my parents' welfare as I would have wished, but there is no reason why I must do what I intended. I am a fallible human being who failed on this occasion, but I am not damnable.'

When you feel remorse, but not guilt, about failing to live up to your standards in some way, you tend to take responsibility for your behaviour without damning your 'self', and you try to understand why you failed to meet the standards you voluntarily embraced. If your parents complain about the pain you 'caused' them through your lack of devotion, you may choose to apologize to them for your lapse, but not to the extent of getting down on your knees and desperately pleading for their forgiveness.

If you have worked hard with the exercises outlined in this chapter so far, and have rid yourself of the iBs concerning your need for your parents' approval, or being responsible for unstintingly devoting yourself to them, you are now ready to go on to Key Task No. 2. However, make sure that you really have accomplished Key Task No. 1 before you proceed to Key Task No. 2 If you are not quite sure, practise the exercises again and again and re-read previous chapters until you feel confident that you understand the A–B–C model of emotional disturbance and how to uproot the iBs that sustain it. Only then will you be able to extract the maximum benefit from the remaining two Key Tasks.

Key Task No. 2: Understanding and accepting your parents with their difficult traits and behaviour

This can partly be done by looking at Peter's situation.

Peter understood that his parents' beliefs and attitudes didn't just happen. By reminding himself of the REBT Insights he had gained through his hard work, Peter realized that the beliefs and attitudes currently held by his parents had been acquired over their lifetime, and largely governed and explained their present behaviour. Moreover, Peter was also aware that some kinds of behaviour exhibited by difficult parents may simply result from ignorance or emotional disturbance and, perhaps less commonly, from some kind of deficiency or deficit.

Armed with these insights, Peter made it his first task to get onto his parents' wavelength and to try to communicate a genuine desire to understand their beliefs, hopes, desires and fears. Peter also had a fairly clear idea about the iBs his parents must be holding to account for their over-protective attitude towards him, but he wisely resisted the temptation to confront his parents with their iBs because he realized that such a move would be counterproductive. He will do much better by being a receptive listener right from the start. If we want to understand our parents, it makes good sense to listen to them first!

Receptive listening means listening attentively without reacting negatively or jumping in with *your* opinions. Your aim at this stage is to get inside their world, to see things from their frame of reference. Try to listen to your parents in such a way that you understand the feelings beneath the words and can see what they are thinking and feeling from their point of view. From time to time you can check that your understanding is correct by feeding back to your parents the gist of what you believe they are thinking and feeling. For example, from time to time Peter would gently break in by inquiring. 'Am I right in taking it that you feel shut out when I mention my intention to move out and live on my own somewhere?' Or he would occasionally convey that he understood how his parents felt by saying, 'Yes, I can see now how you feel that way. I guess if I was in your shoes, I would feel exactly the same way.'

Try to talk to your parents, as Peter did, in a gentle, enquiring, non-critical manner. Try to understand their point of view rather than criticize it; don't adopt an adversarial attitude. Make allowances for the powerful influences of the past. In their youth, maybe your parents were taught by their parents and teachers the virtue of self-sacrifice, of living their life for the benefit of others, of putting the welfare of their children or the common good above their own personal interests, and so on. Make allowances for the powerful influence of the social roles and cultural norms to which your parents and their forebears were exposed during their impressionable years, and the societal models people were expected to follow. Although today these traditional roles are being increasingly questioned and challenged, traditional role models still exercise a considerable influence over people. So don't expect your parents to give up their long-held views overnight that they exist mainly for your sake, or that it is your duty to look after them. If you show them that you understand their views and that you appreciate that their efforts over the years were motivated by a genuine concern for your welfare, you may make it easier for them eventually to accept that your desire for a greater degree of independence does not in any way imply criticism of them personally for the way they brought you up.

Empathic listening doesn't mean that you have to agree with everything your parents assert about how you should live your life. Empathic listening simply gives them the opportunity to be heard fully, to be listened to, and to know that their feelings have been understood. Once they know that you have understood and appreciated

57

their point of view, they are less likely to try to impose their views upon you.

Once you have succeeded in conveying to your parents that you understand why they brought you up in the way they did, it is important to show them that you accept that they had the right to do what they thought was correct at the time. Sensibly, that was the strategy Peter adopted. Peter saw that the real issue was not whether he loved his parents. Peter loved his parents and he knew that they loved him. The real issue was not love, but the kind and degree of love that would be compatible with the healthy measure of personal independence and autonomy that Peter sought to attain. If that is your goal, you can show your parents that you can see that they acted as any good parents would have done, given the information on child upbringing available to them at the time. If you put your parents down for not having treated you as you would treat a young person growing into adulthood today, you will feel angry and resentful. And if you put yourself down for feeling angry and resentful, guilt and/or depression may result. Since you know by now how unhelpful these negative emotions can be to those who experience them, you will readily see that it makes good sense to accept yourself and other people unconditionally.

Far from accusing your parents of having over-protected you, you can point out how grateful you are for having parents who really cared about you. If they are now being asked to take something of a back seat and retire gracefully, that is because you have now reached that stage in your life when you can mature as an individual adult person only by achieving a measure of independence and making your own decisions.

If you can train yourself to converse with your parents in a manner that conveys warmth, understanding and respect for their right to their views (whether you agree with them or not), then your non-blaming and accepting attitude may eventually encourage them to become less fearful of losing you, and to respond more positively to your constructive attempts to create a healthier kind of loving relationship with them.

Key Task No. 3: Acting in an enlightened self-interested way towards your parents

At the same time as Peter was attempting to create a closer understanding between himself and his parents, he continued to show his parents that he accepted them regardless of whether they agreed with his views, and regardless of whether they changed their own views. He conveyed to his parents that they need have no fears that he was about to abandon them, and that what he was seeking was actually a closer, more adult relationship with his parents, based not on too much dependence of one party upon the other, but upon a mutual recognition of the right of each person to his or her freedom and independence to live their life as fully as their circumstances permit. Peter conveyed clearly to his parents that he still valued their love and affection and that he wanted it to continue, but that it would bring more satisfaction to all three of them if that mutuality of feeling was shared on a freely given basis of equality, rather than on a perception that it was a filial or parental duty.

Old habits need time to wither away

We would caution you not to expect your parents to relinquish their old habits of relating to you overnight. They will find it requires quite an effort on their part to change, to reorientate their thinking. Perhaps they won't change at all, or perhaps they may change a little bit – but not feel too happy about it. Don't upset yourself about it! Continue to listen to their views and show your parents that you understand and accept them.

Resist the temptation to argue when you and they hold differing views. If you disagree with them, and they invite you to explain yourself, patiently and politely explain why you cannot accept their viewpoint, but refrain from condemning or criticizing. Avoid 'you' statements, such as, 'You're wrong about that'; instead, use 'I' statements, such as, 'My own view is . . . ?', or 'I happen to believe that . . .'.

Explain how parents and their adult offspring can be interdependent and help one another in mutually acceptable ways without necessarily infringing each other's individual independence or autonomy. Show by example that nobody is obligated to live their life for someone else's benefit. You may *choose* to sacrifice a large measure of your own independence to look after a sick or elderly parent or relative for example, but it is your choice. You're not here to live your life for the benefit of others. It may take time for these ideas to sink in. But when they do, your relationship with your parents could improve in a way you previously would not have believed possible.

With patience and understanding coupled with perseverance, you can make progress. Help your parents to realize that you putting your own interests first does not mean that you have become less loving, or that you intend to neglect them in the future. You can state your view that genuine love depends upon freedom; you cannot coerce someone to love you. If the issue of selfishness comes up, you can explain that in your view, putting your own interests first is not being selfish, but that demanding that others put your interests first *is* being selfish!

Love between you and your parents can grow, rather than shrink, as in time you come to a better mutual understanding and regard for one another's personal freedom and autonomy. However, that is unlikely to happen if you allow the seeds of your emerging new, more mature kind of love to be trampled under in the name of duty, self-sacrifice or social responsibility.

The importance of striking a balance

As we have stated, acting in an enlightened self-interested way towards your parents involves striking a balance between your own short-term and long-term goals and the interests of others (particularly your parents or significant others).

We cannot tell you where to draw the line between acting in your own best interests and giving up your time to promote the welfare of your parents. That must be your decision. Each situation is different and is best judged on its merits. In Peter's case, his task was relatively easy. His parents didn't demand his unstinting devotion to their welfare. The problem lay mainly with Peter himself. Once Peter had truly convinced himself that he didn't have to have his parents' approval for the way he wanted to run his own life and no longer felt ashamed when he incurred their disapproval, he was able to take the first steps to severing his over-dependence upon their approval and to lead a more independent life. Eventually, Peter did leave his parents' home and lived successfully in a flat of his own.

By contrast, if you find yourself with very dependent parents for whose sake you have given up a good deal of your own time to look after their interests at the expense of your own, your problem is to decide just how far you are prepared to go in sacrificing yourself for your parents.

The main factors to be taken into consideration would include the degree of disablement (if any) that applies to them, their age and general health, what coping skills they have acquired, and the degree to which the social and/or medical services are currently involved, or might be required later. You also need to assess your own long- and short-term goals, and how far these could be compromised should you decide to undertake the role of care-giver and all that it implies. Altogether, not an easy calculation to make!

Be honest with yourself and others; don't hide behind a cardboard cutout of yourself and pretend to be something you are not. To reveal your true desires and opinions sometimes takes courage. You have to be willing to accept the disapproval – even the condemnation – of others that may follow the honest exposure of your interests and values. Take heart! Other people's words and attitudes can't hurt you unless you take them seriously.

It takes time to know yourself, to throw off a lifetime of pressures to sacrifice yourself for this, or for that, and just to relax and accept yourself no matter how your views may conflict with prevailing social standards, and to act in ways consistent with your nature. One of the consequences you will experience when you are being honest with people and acting sincerely towards them is that you attract those who admire what you stand for. If your parents learn to accept and trust you, they may eventually come to admire and love you not because of how you used to sacrifice yourself for them, but because of who you are. Only then will you and your parents be free to enjoy the honest expression of mutually shared feelings, and even to love each other without loving 'too much'.

4

How to Cope with Rejecting
and Neglectful Parents

In the previous chapter, we showed you how to love your parents without loving them 'too much'; in this chapter, we look at the other side of the coin. We deal here with the problems that may arise if you were brought up by parents whom you considered didn't love you enough: parents who neglected and rejected you when you were a child in their care, and still continue to do so. There are various kinds and degrees of rejection and neglect, but we will not be concerning ourselves with that aspect of the matter. Our main concern here is to show you how to cope with rejection and neglect, regardless of what form it takes.

Parents who reject and neglect their children may do so for a variety of reasons. You will recall that on page 22 we listed three main reasons for parents' difficult behaviour: (i) ignorance; (ii) emotional disturbance; (iii) deficiency. (Re-read page 22 again if you need to.) We consider that within these three categories can be found the great majority of the reasons for parents' poor upbringing of their children.

We will start by looking at how 'survivors' of poor parental upbringing think and feel about their early upbringing, and how they are coping today with parents who still behave towards their adult offspring in rejecting and neglectful ways.

If you were brought up by parents who often rejected or neglected you when you were a child and who still show no signs of wanting to move to a closer or warmer relationship with you now that you are grown up, you may not really care that much, especially if you have little or no contact with them now, and have no intention of doing anything different in the future. If this is the case, then you can skip this chapter.

However, if you still maintain contact with your parents to some degree, and you would like to learn how to cope with them without upsetting yourself over the way they often treated you as a child, or over their continuing lack of warmth or interest in you, then the rest of this chapter will provide you with the necessary insights and understanding to achieve your goal.

Some typical kinds of parental rejection and neglect

Every survivor of 'troubled' families has their own individual story to tell. It is important, though, to bear in mind that you are given only one side of the story – the parents are not usually invited to give their side.

As a child, you were totally dependent upon your parents or parent substitutes for your physical and emotional well-being. No parents are perfect, of course, and even the best parents will make mistakes. But generally speaking, parents are aware of their responsibilities towards their children, and do their best with the resources at their disposal to give their children a decent upbringing, in all its many facets.

By contrast, if you grew up in a severely troubled family and your need for love and care was largely unfulfilled, you were probably too young to understand the reasons behind your parents' rejection and lack of interest in you. If you were trapped in an environment marked, for example, by bouts of alcoholism, and occasional outbursts of bitter fighting or physical abuse of one parent by the other, you probably felt frightened, apprehensive and insecure. And as you grew up, you were aware mainly of the chronic lack of fulfilment of your own emotional needs. When you went to your parents for affection you were pushed away; they never seemed to have time for you. As a result, your natural healthy desires and needs to feel loved and to share your own feelings with someone you felt close to were not met. You can recall many times when you were ignored, told to go away, and not to be so troublesome. Sometimes you recall being pushed away with a 'Don't bother me now'.

Here are a few of the ways in which you might have experienced rejection and neglect as you grew up from childhood to adolescence.

Perhaps mealtimes were irregular, and often lacking in quality and/or quantity. Or you may have been physically neglected and left alone for long periods, or in the care of some neighbour or relative. Your dental health and general physical well-being may have been neglected because your parents never bothered to take you to the doctor or dentist for regular check-ups. Your accomplishments at school possibly went largely unrecognized by your parents. You seldom received a word of praise or encouragement for anything you did well – perhaps you are hard put to recall a single instance of your parents singing your praises or showing approval.

Later, as you reached adolescence, your right to privacy may frequently have been disrespected or invaded. No room in the house was ever one that you could call your own; even your personal belongings were frequently removed or used without your permission. Perhaps when you reached adolescence, there were times when your parents tried to involve you in their quarrels, which each parent trying to enlist you on his or her side against the other, with you feeling like the helpless 'pig in the middle'.

Communication between you and your parents may have been severely restricted, with not much talk about feelings. Normal conversation consisted mainly of checking up on whether you had done your homework, and whether you had carried out all those other parental instructions you received almost daily. If you had some personal problem, an even greater problem was knowing which parent you could approach to discuss it with. Usually, you either were not really listened to, or you were unceremoniously squashed and told to shut up.

It's unlikely you experienced all of these disadvantages, but you might have experienced some of them. However, it is important to note that as as child, you had a natural tendency to take everything too seriously. You lacked the ability to make adequate discriminations between the reasons behind all the things you were told to do and not to do. Consequently, by the time you had grown up, you felt that the clear unmistakable message you had been receiving from your parents throughout your life was simply: your feelings are of little account, or your feelings are your own business.

As a result, you may have come to see yourself as you grew up as a helpless victim of your past, unable ever to get over those hurtful, belittling experiences etched so vividly into the memories of your childhood and later years. In the following pages, we will attempt to show you how to avoid falling into the trap of seeing yourself as a powerless 'victim', and how to acquire the skills to cope with your parents' present behaviour.

You are not a victim

You cannot undo the past: nor can you change your parents. However, you *can* change the way you view your past, and you can undo the negative view of yourself that you may have developed. That came about partly as a result of your becoming emotionally disturbed over the way your parents and maybe others in your family or social group treated you during your vulnerable childhood years. We need to make it clear here that we are certainly not condoning your parents' behaviour; unquestionably, your parents contributed to your upset feelings. For some reason they were unable to let themselves relate to you in the naturally loving, caring way that characterizes healthy parent–child relationships. However, your principal concern at this stage is to understand that your parents didn't *make* you upset. No doubt they went the right way about trying to upset you, but that was *their* problem, and we shall discuss that later.

Right now we want to help you see that the main reason you upset yourself when you were a child was partly because you were born 'disturbable' in the first place. We believe that humans have an inborn tendency to think irrationally, as well as rationally, and that our emotions and behaviour are influenced by these biological tendencies in addition to the influences of education, upbringing and environmental conditions to which we are exposed throughout our lives.

As a child, you found it easy to disturb yourself because you listened to and accepted your parents' rejection and neglect of your childhood need for expressed affection, and you drew the seemingly obvious conclusion that you must be unlovable, that there must be something wrong with you. Then you put yourself down. They rejected you by not giving you the love, time or attention you demanded from them, and that felt terrible.

The pain you experienced as a child may well have gone very deep, but that was because you lacked the means to set limits to it. As a child, you were extremely vulnerable to rejection and its implication that you were somehow unworthy of love and attention. The child mind is relatively simple and unsophisticated; it would never have occurred to you that the reason for your rejection and neglect was because there might be something amiss with your parents!

However, now you are an adult, and you can handle rejection and neglect because you have the resources you need to understand how you upset yourself in the past and how to use that understanding to overcome any present tendency you may have to re-experience the miseries you suffered in the past. So let's make a start by showing you how to use these resources to dump the miseries of your past and give yourself leeway to create a happier future. As in previous chapters, we will structure our discussion of the problem around the Three Key Tasks.

Key Task No 1: Getting yourself into a healthy frame of mind emotionally

If you intend to have some degree of contact with your difficult parents during your adult years, and if you would prefer to get on with them reasonably well, it is important to get yourself into the right frame of mind. As with previous examples, this means acquiring an attitude that will allow you to communicate with them in a non-blaming, non-self-pitying and assertive manner. If you allow yourself to dwell too much on the past and try to 'put the record straight' or to 'get even' with your parents by blaming them for their shortcomings and failures as you compulsively rehash the pain and emotional deprivation you claim you suffered in your youth through their incompetent upbringing, you will succeed only in repeating the past and keeping its miseries alive indefinitely. The past has no magic ability to keep itself alive; you are not destined to repeat it, but you will repeat it if you continue to act as if you were still living in it!

Also, you are likely to succeed in driving your parents away from any contact whatever with you if you keep on and on at them about what a terrible job they made of bringing you up. This is because it is very unlikely that your parents look back upon the period in which they brought you up in quite the same way as you do. Even if your account of your bad upbringing were only *partially* true (and of course we assume that you were not making it up), it is quite possible that your parents may have been somewhat emotionally disturbed themselves, or they may have been so preoccupied with their own problems at the time that they hardly gave a thought to how you felt about yours. (We will go into this side of the matter in more detail when we come to Key Task No. 2.)

Meanwhile, let's focus on the present, and on what you can do to identify and overcome any unconstructive negative reactions you may have that are blocking you from getting on better with your (presumably) still rejecting and neglectful parents.

Let it go!

As we've just said, the past doesn't magically keep itself alive. If you are still upset about what happened to you in your past, it is because you still keep the past alive by continually thinking about it and reminding yourself of how 'terrible' it was. If you still feel emotionally upset over the way you were brought up, it is not because of what happened to you then. Your upset feelings stem from the way you are *now*, in the present, reacting to the memory of your poor upbringing.

To remind yourself of this important point, refer back to Chapter 1, pages 20–21, and re-read the section headed '*Letting go of the past*' (up to and including REBT Insight No. 2). We shall now illustrate the points we have been emphasizing by taking you through the case of Julie.

Introducing Julie

Julie was an only child, who was considered bright for her age and a good pupil at school. The impression that most people had of Julie's parents was of a couple who attached importance to keeping up appearances, and who came across as considerate but somewhat reserved. They never showed any emotion in public, but they did socialize to the extent of being known as regular bridge players and they maintained church connections in their local community.

By the time Julie had reached young adulthood, she viewed her childhood and adolescence as a barren emotional wasteland. Although she was neglected to some extent by her parents, it was a fairly benign form of neglect, and she didn't consider herself to have been unduly harmed by it. In fact, Julie recalled that she received more affection from the parents of her school friends who looked after her during her parents' occasional absences than she ever received from her own parents. What Julie really felt upset about was her parents' chronic lack of affection towards her; apparently they never showed their daughter any overt affection. If she asked for it, even pleaded for it, the result was the same. Whenever Julie went up to her father for an affectionate hug, he would push her away, and her mother would say to her, 'Behave yourself, Julie! You must try to grow up to be a little lady, not a little daddy's girl.' If Julie wanted a little affection from her mother and tried to put an arm around her mother's neck, her mother would pull herself free and push Julie back with a 'Come now, Julie! Remember you're a little girl now, not a little baby.'

Julie's mother attached great importance to decorum, and Julie would recall how the kind of comfortable clothes that she (Julie) preferred to wear, or chose to buy, were often described as 'unsuitable for a young lady' and had to be replaced by garments her mother considered more 'suitable'.

As she grew up, Julie's feelings towards her parents were a mixture of hurt and anger. She felt that she loved her parents – or rather, that she *could* love them, if only they would drop their defences and give her the love and affection she so strongly craved, and which she considered they *should* give.

With her feeling of angry hurt following her constant rejection still unresolved, Julie grew up and eventually got a secretarial job in the town where she lived. Then, much against her parents' wishes, Julie left her parents' home and went to live with Nick, a man whom she had met at work. The relationship didn't last long. Nick resembled Julie's father: he was good-looking, but also reserved and undemonstrative. Julie convinced herself that Nick just needed to be shown love and encouraged to 'open up', and then all would be well. So Julie set about trying to change Nick. Without realizing it, Julie was trying to solve her childhood desire of getting her father to be more like she wanted him to be by picking a man who treated her as her father did, and then trying to change him. It didn't work. When Julie realized she was pregnant, she split up with Nick and returned to live with her parents in the hope that they would now give her the love and support she had been denied over the years she had been in their care. When the support she wished for was not given, Julie's old feelings of hurt and anger came surging back with increased intensity.

The real cause of Julie's anger and hurt

First, Julie inferred that her parents had acted towards her in an 'unfair' manner. They disregarded her desires to be treated in a loving, caring manner, and acted towards her in what to Julie seemed a non-caring way. Other girls seemed to have parents who gave out lots of love and affection, but not Julie's parents. Julie thought this was very unfair, and considered herself undeserving of such treatment.

These inferences alone did not cause Julie to feel hurt and angry. What do you think were Julie's beliefs about her parents' inferred lack of love for her? You will know by now that upset feelings don't arise as a direct result of unfortunate events or circumstances that confront you. Rather, they stem from a number of iBs that you hold about the unfortunate events or circumstances. These iBs of Julie's can be summarized under Major Irrational Belief No. 2.

Major Irrational Belief No. 2

'Because it is preferable that others treat me considerately and fairly, they absolutely should and must; and they are rotten people who deserve to be utterly damned when they do not.'

Julie's feelings of hurt and anger resulted from what she believed about her parents' rejection of her:

- 'My parents absolutely should not have treated me in this unfair manner in the past, nor should they continue to do so. It's terrible to be treated in this way and my parents are no good for treating me like that.'

Now, let's apply the Disputing techniques you have learned to see why Julie's beliefs are irrational.

Disputing Julie's iBs

We will now look at Julie's iBs about the way her parents treated her in the past, and continue to treat her.

(a) *Is this belief logical?* No. Julie may wish that her parents had not treated her in an unfair manner in the past and that they did not still continue to do so, but it doesn't follow that they have to treat Julie as she wishes to be treated.

Nor does it logically follow that because it is unfortunate to be treated in a non-caring manner, it is therefore terrible to be treated in that way.

Also, it does not logically follow that, because Julie's parents may have treated her unfairly and uncaringly in the past and continue to do so, that they are no good at all for treating her in that way. That is an arbitrary value judgement on Julie's part.

(b) *Is this belief consistent with reality?* It is not, for the following reasons: things are exactly what they are at any given moment, and it makes no sense to demand that they should be other than what they are. Since Julie's parents deprived her of the love and consideration she wanted as a child, and still continue to withhold their love, it does not make sense to contend that what happened absolutely should not have happened.

It may have been bad, meaning unfortunate, to be treated with little or no demonstrable affection, but Julie's conviction that it was 'terrible' is a gross over-generalization. To condemn her parents as no good because some of their *acts* were mistaken and unhelpful, is to imply that they as persons were no good, and is therefore also a gross over-generalization. Like all humans, Julie's parents are fallible beings who frequently do wrong things or behave inadequately from time to time. That is the way they are.

(c) *Will this belief help Julie to achieve her goals?* It is highly unlikely! So long as Julie turns her face against accepting her parents with their inadequacies and keeps alive her belief that they absolutely should not have treated her badly, she will be unable to relax and calm down enough to learn from her past. She will fail to see exactly the iBs with which she disturbed herself in the past, and how her present hurt and resentment stem from that same pattern of irrational thinking.

The likely outcome is that Julie risks driving a permanent wedge between herself and her parents at a time when she could benefit greatly from any help she could get from them, quite apart from the advantages that would accrue from finding ways of getting along with her parents in a more amicable manner.

Eventually, Julie saw how unhelpful her iBs were, and that she would continue to feel emotionally upset as long as she held on to them. As we have seen, iBs don't die quickly or easily; you have to work and practise at Disputing them until you really convince yourself that they no longer control your thinking. Yet the more vigorously you Dispute and act against your iBs, the sooner they will lose their grip on you and the sooner you will be able to replace them with more rational alternative beliefs.

After much hard work, Julie finally rid herself of her long-held iB that her parents should not have treated her in the way they did, that it was terrible that they did, and that they were no good. Julie also saw that her present miseries stemmed from that same irrational demand. As a result of her hard work, Julie come to hold a more rational view of her situation.

Julie's rational alternative beliefs

- 'I don't like the way my parents treated me as a child, and I wish they had been more loving towards me, but there is no reason why they shouldn't have acted the way they did, nor is there any reason why they should treat me more lovingly now, although I would definitely prefer them to.

  My parents responded to what was going on in their heads at the time, and they still do. While I felt deprived to some extent by not being given the natural love and affection I wanted when I was a child, it was a disadvantage – not a catastrophe. It makes no sense to condemn them for their mistakes or inadequacies; my parents are fallible human beings, not perfect angels. They made mistakes, as we all do, but they are not bad people and there is no reason why I cannot treat them fairly and considerately, now and in the future.'

Julie's new healthier feelings about her parents

Julie's new rBs led her to experience healthier feelings. She lost her old feelings of hurt and anger over her parents' rejection and neglect when she was a child, although she still felt disappointed at their apparent continuing lack of support for both her and her daughter now that she was a single parent.

At the same time, Julie saw the sense of letting go of the past, of giving up squandering her energy on endless 'awfulizing' about the 'unfairness' of her upbringing, and instead decided to direct her efforts to creating a happier life for herself and her daughter both in the present and in the future. Julie was not prepared to forget the past or the pain she suffered as a child when her parents rejected her, but with her more rational frame of mind she felt able to understand and forgive her parents.

You can learn from the past. Here are some important lessons to remember if you had parents who rejected and neglected you when you were a child and who still continue to do so:

- If your parents treated you badly in the past and still continue to reject and neglect you, they have definitely contributed to your anguish, but they haven't *caused* it. The reason you originally became upset was your 'musts', 'shoulds' and 'oughts' about their behaviour towards you.

- If you are still feeling upset today, it is because you are still holding on to these 'musts', 'shoulds' and 'oughts' with which you upset yourself originally.

- It may even be appealing to refuse to face up to your own part in creating your early emotional miseries and instead to accept the status of 'victim'. People will feel sorry for you and sympathize with you; but if this happens, you will never grow up. You will always be a baby, whining about the injustices of the past, and why your past miseries account for your unhappiness now.

It's so easy to blame the past because you can then avoid taking responsibility for failing to see what you are doing to maintain these childhood upsets in your present. The result is that you condemn yourself to living in the past and sabotage your potential for living more enjoyably in the present.

Let's turn now to Key Task No. 2 to discover how Julie's more rational attitude towards her parents helped her to understand and accept them.

Key Task No. 2: Understanding and accepting your parents with their difficult traits and behaviour

In previous chapters we have explained why it is important to understand and accept your parents if you want to improve your relationship with them, so we won't waste time repeating ourselves, but instead we will deal directly with how to go about your task – using the case of Julie as an example.

Understanding your parents involves seeing the world from their perspective. How did they feel about you and how did they come to be the way they were? As a young child, you probably didn't understand much about what was going on in your parents' lives. Later on, as you reached adolescence and entered your teens, you probably had a fair idea of what your working parent did for a living, and whether your parents' personal relationship was relatively harmonious. In Julie's case, her father worked for a firm of accountants and the family were fairly well off. Julie recalled that she never saw her parents display any open affection to one another. Neither of them ever gave the other an affectionate hug or kiss, or at least never in Julie's presence. As Julie wryly observed, 'At least my parents acted consistently. They just didn't seem to believe in showing their feelings, not even to each other. I often used to wonder if they really had any feelings!'

Now able to look at her parents' behaviour from an adult perspective and from a more rational point of view, Julie began to realize that her parents probably had problems she was totally unaware of when she was a child in their care. Julie would have liked her parents to show her more affection, but she realized now that their apparent inability to express love or affection did not mean that there was something intrinsically unlovable about her. She recalled that she never went without adequate food or clothing; the house they lived in was comfortable and warm. Although there were times when she was neglected, her parents never left her on her own, or with neighbours, for very long periods. To Julie, they seemed long at the time, but she now realized that a child's perception of time is different from that of an adult.

Thus Julie realized that her feelings of angry hurt in the past stemmed from iBs that she acquired in the past, and that these same iBs still dominated her thinking in the present. That explained why she still felt hurt and angry at her parents' continuing rejection and neglect. Similarly, Julie saw that her parents' rejection and neglect of her emotional needs in the past probably stemmed from iBs they had picked up that effectively inhibited them from displaying emotion – iBs that evidently still dominated their thinking, and therefore their feelings and behaviour, towards Julie today.

Julie also admitted to her parents her own part in creating the many emotional upsets she experienced as a child. She explained that as a child she tended to take everything too seriously, as children naturally do, and that she easily upset herself over matters that her parents saw as minor irritations. Julie also accepted responsibility for having continued to upset herself after she had grown up, not only about her traumas over her parents' rejection of her desire for love in the past, but also over their continuing rejection of her overtures in the present. As Julie put it, 'I still continued to view my parents and the events of my childhood through the eyes of a child.'

Once you have conveyed to your parents that you understand and appreciate their viewpoint and that you feel affection for them (assuming that you do), your task is to show your parents that you accept them. Let's go on to show you what that means.

As we have seen, accepting your parents means taking them as they are without necessarily liking what they do. Now take Julie as an example again. As she surveyed her situation, she was pleased to see how she had helped herself to get over her hurt and anger towards her parents by abandoning her iB that it was terrible that her parents withheld their love from her and that this 'made' her feel a reject. She no longer put her parents down for not giving her the love and affection she had demanded in the past; Julie accepted that her parents are human too. They also had been taught iBs about themselves and the world they lived in, just as she had. She saw that her task now was to accept that they also had a right to their beliefs, to make mistakes, and to bring their child up in whatever way they thought was right at the time – without being blamed or condemned for being rigid about dress codes and inhibited about the expression of feelings. That did not, of course, imply condoning their behaviour. Julie accepted her parents, not their rejecting and neglectful deeds.

So given Julie's parents' background and the somewhat rigid ideas they had about bringing her up, does it make sense to expect them to have treated her differently? Does it make sense to expect them suddenly to change and behave any differently towards her now? And what possible advantage would Julie get by blaming them and ostracizing them now for their past and present shortcomings?

If your parents are like Julie's, you may think it a good idea to perform little acts that show kindness or affection for your parents, whether or not your acts are reciprocated; and you can demonstrate, as Julie did through giving her own daughter lots of openly expressed love and affection in her grandparents' presence, that such behaviour is normal and natural. Whether your clear acceptance of your parents, together with your own unabashed display of affection in their presence, will encourage your parents to 'open up' is difficult to say; at the very least, it won't do any harm. It's possible that they may never overcome their blocks to expressing emotion. You may be disappointed, but you need not anger yourself, or put yourself or them down in any way whatsoever.

Demonstrating understanding and acceptance of your parents and showing willingness to work towards creating a more agreeable and sustainable relationship with them in the future will provide a better basis for achieving it than condemning them for their rejection and neglect in the past and/or in the present.

Key Task No. 3: Acting in an enlightened self-interested way towards your parents

It is useful at the outset to have as clear an idea as you can of the extent to which you are willing to involve yourself in your parents' life, and it is equally important to know how far they wish to become involved in yours. Rejecting and neglecting parents may desire only minimal contact with their adult offspring. If this is your experience, you may be tempted to compensate by trying to get too involved in your parents' life. You can accept your parents with their rejection and neglect, but you don't have to put up with too much of it. You can set limits to what you are willing to tolerate. If their rejection is total, then obviously no relationship is possible. However, if they only balk at openly expressing affection towards you, or your children, there is no reason why you and they cannot live with it. You don't have to like it, but you can tolerate it.

There's a balance to be sought between being too much involved and not involved enough. That is why it is important to decide where your priorities lie, to identify your short- and long-term goals, and to distinguish your primary interests from those of lesser significance. Where do your parents' interests fit in? Are they of primary importance to you, or can they be put in the box marked 'lesser importance'? Since only you know what you want to do with your life, only you can make those decisions. Here, it is important for you to communicate to your parents your needs and desires and to invite them to express theirs. Do you wish to spend more time together, to have your parents take more interest in you and/or your children? If so, give them the opportunity, but don't demand that they take it up.

Julie decided to take the initiative. She invited her parents to spend time with her and her daughter. She encouraged her parents to play with their granddaughter in the local park, put her on the swings and roundabouts, and generally establish a bond with their grandchild. Julie praised her parents when they took the initiative and shared moments of fun and laughter with the child. Through her personal example, Julie showed her parents how to relax and 'let their hair down', and how much more satisfying life could be by getting involved in it instead of observing it from the sidelines. Julie's unabashed and frequent displays of affection towards her daughter conveyed to her parents the idea that it isn't shameful or a sign of weakness to display one's feelings in public. As time went by, Julie's parents seemed to 'lighten up' a bit, and eventually, at Julie's suggestion, they took their granddaughter out at regular intervals to various public places where she could play under their supervision. Gradually, Julie's parents began to perform little services for Julie and her daughter. They expressed their pleasure at being together on several occasions, and although they never became highly demonstrative, they lost some of their reserve and seemed happy to give, and eventually to receive, occasional expressions of affection from Julie and their granddaugher.

Not every case of parental rejection and neglect will have this relatively happy outcome. Some individuals may never change their ways. So be it; you can't change people against their will. However, once your parents know that their views are understood and appreciated and that you accept them without necessarily going along with their ideas and values, you may be able to help them to become more actively involved with you by enlarging their conceptions of what life is about. You can show your parents what life has to offer them now in the way of new experiences, new interests, new opportunities. Even if you achieve only a modest success in expanding their horizons, you may find that the improvement in the quality of your relationship with them was well worth your time and effort.

5

How to Cope with Demanding and Critical Parents

If you have ever been on the receiving end of carping criticism that just goes on and on, or if you have ever been subjected to demands that never seem to stop, then you will know all too well what this feels like. Some 'demanders' are never satisfied, while others seem to desire to do nothing else in life except criticize their nearest (but alas, no longer dearest). It seems to be a way of life with such people. If they had nobody to criticize continually or make demands upon, they would be completely lost for something to do.

We cannot stop parents from constantly criticizing you or persuade them to become less demanding, but once you show them that you are no longer so easily upset by the constant criticism and complaint, it's possible that they might begin to change their ways. Our aim in writing this chapter is to show you ways of handling yourself in these situations so that you don't end up in a fit of violent rage or a mood of sulky resentment and self-pity.

When you were a child, you were probably not so much criticized as corrected. You were told what to do and what not to do. If you did the wrong thing, as doubtless you did on many occasions, you were corrected – and possibly also penalized or punished in some way. If your parents or guardians caught you playing with a dangerous implement, they simply took it away from you and told you that you mustn't do it again. You gradually learned what behaviour was acceptable and what wasn't.

Later in life, as you entered your teens, criticism replaced correction, and demands were made that you do this or don't do that. Typically, your parents constantly criticized your taste in reading material, the kind of music you listened to, the style of clothes you wore, and the kind of friends you went out with. Then came the demands. You must do your share of the housework, keep your room clean and tidy, hang up your clothes, do your school homework before you switch on the television, be home by a certain time if you went out for the evening, etc.

If you were lucky, the criticism and demands diminished as you became older, and by the time you had reached adulthood, they had virtually ceased. But not always! Largely because of unresolved problems of their own, some parents are unable to let go even when you have grown up and left home and are looking after yourself. The criticism and demanding continues unabated and can seriously impair your relationship with your parents. It is this situation we shall mainly focus our attention upon in this chapter. However, if you are a teenager still living with your parents, you may also find it helpful to study our analysis and follow the advice relevant to your circumstances.

Let's assume that your parents have never really changed, and that over the years the criticism and demands have gone on and on. The kind of things they criticize you for and the kind of demands they make upon you nowadays may have changed, but that's about the only difference. How do you react to this apparently never-ending barrage? Anger is one common reaction. The trouble with anger, as we have already shown, is that it seldom does you any good. The relationship you presently have with your parents may leave a lot to be desired, but getting angry with your parents is more likely to make things worse, not better. So let's look at healthier, more constructive ways of responding to your parents' difficult behaviour with a view to obtaining, if possible, a more mutually agreeable way of getting along together.

Unfortunately, there are many unconstructive responses you can make when trying to deal with critical and demanding parents. Two of the most unhelpful reactions that people typically experience when they are being constantly criticized by demanding parents are feeling hurt and experiencing self-pity. These two negative and unhealthy emotional reactions to over-critical and demanding parents will be the main focus of our attention in this chapter. Feelings of hurt and self-pity tend to block you from taking a rational view of your situation. Not only are the feelings unpleasant or uncomfortable, but also they encourage you to act in various unconstructive ways that do nothing to solve your problem with your parents. For example, a common reaction is to withdraw all communication with your parents (collo-quially referred to as 'sulking'). That kind of reaction will hardly persuade your parents to stop criticizing you. One so-called 'solution' (although it may in the long term prove far from a 'solution') is to escape the parental home by getting married, as the following case study will illustrate.

Introducing Shirley

When Shirley was growing up, she was regarded as the black sheep of the family. Her older sister had become a lawyer, while her younger brother was studying to become an architect. Shirley, on the other hand, had no interest in the professions; she was not academically inclined, and after leaving school she got a job as a waitress in a restaurant.

Shirley had always been the main recipient of her parents' criticism. At school they continually criticized her for not doing well enough, and kept pushing her to do better. Endless comparisons were made between the fine results being achieved by her sister and brother at the end of each term, and the meagre achievements attained by Shirley. 'Lazy little pup' was one of the less demeaning names Shirley was called by her parents, who never tired of telling her that she could do better, and must do better. These demands were often accompanied by predictions of the dire straits in which she would find herself one day if she didn't 'buck up' her ideas and become a credit to her parents, just like her industrious sister and brother.

In addition to their constant demands upon Shirley to do better at school and to work hard at home, Shirley's parents insisted on choosing her friends for her as well as deciding the type of entertainment she was permitted to attend – 'all in her best interests', of course! Everything Shirley enjoyed doing was monitored. The music she listened to, the TV and videos she watched, the magazines she read, all had to receive the golden seal of parental approval.

Later, when she had grown up, Shirley recalled that while her parents tended also to be quite critical and demanding towards her sister and brother at times, she seemed to be singled out for extra attention. By the time Shirley was 20, she decided she had had enough. At her workplace, she met and fell in love with a twice divorced man with two children from a previous marriage. This man never criticized her, and offered a sympathetic ear to Shirley's complaints about her parents' constant nagging and endless demands. Soon they were married.

Shirley's parents were not amused. The air of frosty politeness with which they attended Shirley's wedding hinted ominously at possible repercussions later. Scarcely had Shirley and her husband returned from their honeymoon then Shirley's parents made their presence known. Instead of leaving the couple to get on with their marriage, Shirley's parents made a point of never being far away. They would call round at unexpected and often inconvenient times, brushing aside

Shirley's remonstrations with a 'You surely don't think we're going to abandon our daughter just because she's now married?' Or, one of them would say, 'Beginning married life can be difficult for a young couple these days. I'm sure there must be something we can do to help!' Shirley's parents then began to make suggestions about all sorts of changes they thought Shirley should make in her home, even to the extent of actually rearranging Shirley's dining-room furniture and changing the colour of her curtains to show how much brighter the room would look. Never at a loss for something to criticize, Shirley's parents would make disparaging comments about the clothes she wore at home, and even offered Shirley money to 'go out and buy yourself something decent to put on, seeing that man of yours doesn't seem to care!'

When her mother began to phone her up late at nights, 'just to see how you are, dear', in addition to her parents' frequently unannounced and largely unwelcome visits at weekends, Shirley broke down in tears. First, she felt hard done by because of the way her parents had treated her in the past – always criticizing her for not being good enough, demanding she do this or that, and restricting her desires to do what she wanted to do. Then when she left her parent's home and escaped, or so she thought, from all that interminable criticizing and denigration, only to discover to her dismay that what she had thought she had left behind for good was now re-emerging in an even worse form in her married life, it was hardly surprising that Shirley felt really sorry for herself. Then, to make matters worse, her husband began to blame her for not standing up to her parents and for allowing them to interfere in the marriage. 'Your parents are a blasted pain in the butt!' he told Shirley, and then added, 'And it's all your fault!'

To Shirley, that was the last straw. 'I don't deserve this,' she sobbed. 'Life shouldn't be so unfair and I can't stand it any more!' Shirley's self-pity came from her belief that 'life should be easy and fair and go the way I want. Since it doesn't, it's awful and I can't stand it, and I'll never know happiness again.'

Now, piecing together all that you know about Shirley so far, what iBs would Shirley be holding to account for her feeling of self-pity? You already have been given a clue from her belief that life should be easy and fair.

Shirley's iBs

Expressed in full, Shirley's basic iB about her situation vis-á-vis her parents is:

- 'My parents absolutely should treat me better than they do; and if they continue to criticize and harass me, and cause needless problems and hassles for me and my husband, they're awful and horrible; and I can't stand the difficulties and unfairness they are creating, and life is hardly worth living!'

This particular iB is a variant of yet another Major Irrational Belief (No.3):

Major Irrational Belief No.3
'My life conditions must give me the things I want and have to have to feel safe and comfortable or else life is unbearable and I can't be happy at all!'

It is important to realize that people who adhere to Major Irrational Belief No.3 hold a philosophy of Low Frustration Tolerance or LFT. Such people believe that they must be comfortable, and thus avoid working to bring about change in their lives because such work inevitably involves experiencing discomfort and inconvenience. In other words, LFT is a philosophy or a personal rule that states, in effect, 'I shouldn't have to do anything that is unpleasant or uncomfortable even if it would be in my best long-term interests. I'd sooner maintain the status quo than risk discomfort.'

Observe how the demands in Major Irrational Belief No.3 lead to procrastination, poor self-discipline and – when these demands are not met – to feelings of self-pity, and could – if not vigorously Disputed – lead into feelings of helplessness, hopelessness and ultimately depression.

You have now been introduced to the two main categories into which we can put virtually all emotional problems; we call them (1) Ego Disturbance (or self-downing), and (2) Discomfort Disturbance (or Low Frustration Tolerance (LFT)). In Chapter 3, Peter's problem with anxiety and shame is an example of Ego Disturbance, while Shirley's problem of self-pity stems from her Low Frustration Tolerance, and falls under the heading of Discomfort Disturbance.

Now you will probably agree that profound feelings of self-pity are not likely to motivate Shirley to take any kind of constructive action to ameliorate her situation. To accomplish that, Shirley will require to change her attitude towards her parents and their difficult behaviour. If she doesn't change, her parents' obnoxious behaviour is likely to continue. To change her self-pitying attitude towards a healthier, more appropriate one is now Shirley's Key Task No. 1.

Key Task No. 1: Getting yourself into a healthy frame of mind emotionally

To change the way she thinks, Shirley will have to examine her presently held iBs and replace them with rational alternatives that can stand up to critical examination. We will now proceed to examine Shirley's statements using the Disputing techniques with which you are now familiar.

Disputing Shirley's iBs

For convenience, we repeat them here:

- 'My parents absolutely should treat me better than they do; and if they continue to criticize and harass me, and cause needless problems and hassles for me and my husband, they are awful and horrible; and I can't stand the difficulties and unfairness they are creating, and life is hardly worth living!'

(a) *Is this belief logical?* No. Shirley obviously wants her parents to treat her better than they do, but does it logically follow that they must? No matter how much we may desire something, it doesn't follow that we absolutely have to get it.

Shirley believes her parents are awful and horrible if they continue to criticize and harass her. Granted, it may be unpleasant and unhelpful if her parents continue to criticize and harass her, but it does not logically follow that her parents become awful and horrible. That is a gross over-generalization, and also represents an arbitrary value judgement on Shirley's part.

Shirley's conclusion that she can't stand a continuation of her parents' critical behaviour because she finds it unpleasant makes no logical sense. You may dislike something, but the fact that you dislike it does not necessarily imply that you cannot stand it.

Lastly, Shirley believes that if her parents continue with their criticisms and demands, then her life is no longer worth living. This may be her own personal definition of her situation, but it does not logically follow that even if her situation is unpleasant, then she can never be happy again.

81

Thus, not a single one of Shirley's contentions has any logical validity. We now proceed to see if her belief is in accord with reality.

(b) *Is this belief consistent with reality?* Far from it! If there were some law that laid it down that Shirley's parents absolutely must treat her better than they do, then she would be treated better. The statement is actually self-contradictory because it is saying that her parents are not now treating her as they absolutely should.

Next, the words 'awful' and 'horrible' really mean not just bad or very bad, but 101 per cent bad. Since nothing can be more than 100 per cent bad, the statement does not correspond with reality. Moreover, it is a gross exaggeration to describe a person as awful or horrible merely on the basis of possessing traits that most people might describe as bad or unfortunate. Also, while you may rate a person's traits, deeds and behaviours, you cannot legitimately confer any kind of global judgement or rating upon the person. Shirley's parents are not, and cannot be, 'awful' or 'horrible', but their behaviour may be mistaken, frustrating and unhelpful.

Finally, nobody – realistically speaking – can predict the future. Therefore Shirley's claim that she can never be happy again makes no sense.

(c) *Does this belief help Shirley to achieve her goals?* It is unlikely. Shirley's goal is to get on with her own life, to make a success of her marriage, and presumably to have a better relationship with her parents through persuading them to be less critical and demanding; and to accept that she has a right to decide, with her husband, how they choose to live their lives – whether or not her parents agree with her decisions.

Shirley's 'poor me' attitude and Low Frustration Tolerance of her parents' over-critical and demanding behaviour will tend to discourage her from looking for constructive ways to solve her problem with her parents, and her denigrating attitude towards her parents will hardly persuade them to change their critical ways. A much better way for Shirley to begin to tackle her problems with her parents would be to acquire 'High Frustration Tolerance' (HFT). She can achieve this – as you will see – by Disputing the iBs that underlie her LFT and replacing them with rational alternative beliefs. This would encourage her to accept (not necessarily like) her parents' difficult behaviour, and would lead to greater patience, and determination to understand her parents and their background with the aim of getting along better with them. That would be Shirley's Key Task No. 2.

Using rational self-statements

In addition to practising her Disputing, Shirley can weaken her iBs by using what we call 'rational self-statements'. She does this by very forcefully repeating to herself 50 times a day the following rational self-statements:

1. 'Nothing is awful or terrible – only inconvenient!'
2. 'I *can* stand what I don't like!'
3. 'No human is damnable and worthless – and that includes both my parents and me!'
4. 'I don't *need* what I want!'

The purpose of this exercise and the persistent and vigorous Disputing of her iBs is to help Shirley to change those core iBs that she has spent her whole life rehearsing, living and 'feeling'. Basically what Shirley is trying to do is to learn new ways of thinking and feeling – ways that will help her to feel better and not be emotionally upset by the behaviour of her parents.

This brings us naturally to REBT Insight No. 3:

REBT Insight No. 3

There is no way other than persistent work and practice to change your iBs, unhealthy feelings and self-destructive behaviours.

You now have been introduced in this and the preceding chapters to the three REBT Insights. Memorize them and use them. Write them down, or type them on a card, so that you can conveniently see them together. Then say them out loud to yourself until you automatically recall them every time you feel angry, depressed or self-pitying. Shirley took our advice; she worked hard at Disputing her iBs and regularly carried out the exercise set out above. As a result of her efforts, Shirley came to hold a more rational set of beliefs about herself and her difficult parents. These were along the following lines:

Shirley's rational alternative beliefs

- 'I would definitely prefer my parents to treat me better, but they don't have to. If they continue to criticize me and harass me, and cause needless problems and hassles for me and my husband, I don't have to find it awful, but merely inconvenient and disadvantageous. Although I'll never like their constant criticism, demands and interference with my marriage, I can certainly stand it. And if they continue to act badly, that only proves they are people with problems, who cannot for the moment treat me as considerately as I'd prefer, but that doesn't make them horrible ogres incapable of ever changing their ways. Even if they don't change their ways, life does not cease to be worth living. By refusing to take life's hassles and difficulties too seriously and turning them into calamities, I can learn to accept my parents with their difficult behaviour and still lead a reasonably happy life.'

As Shirley Disputed her previous iBs and came to see that her new rBs made good sense, she began to look at better ways of responding to her parents' demanding and critical behaviour. The points to be taken here are that once you rid yourself of your self-defeating iBs about the 'unfairness' and the 'horror' of being constantly criticized by your demanding parents, you open up the possibility of solving your problems with your difficult parents in a constructive manner. You then tend to see being criticized, harassed or belittled as a problem to be solved, rather than a catastrophe about which you can do nothing – except to moan and feel sorry for yourself.

To reinforce the techniques of Disputing that you have already learned, and the use of rational self-statements, we are now going to introduce you to another effective method of combating your iBs and developing your 'emotional muscle'; it's called Rational-Emotive Imagery (REI).

How to use Rational-Emotive Imagery (REI) effectively

This method was originated by Dr Maxie C. Maultsby, Jr, a rational-behavioural psychiatrist, and adapted by Dr Albert Ellis for use in REBT. To use REI let us suppose that you have over-critical and demanding parents, just like Shirley, and that they have severely criticized you for some alleged failing. They have given you a particularly difficult time. We shall denote this as **A**, the Activating Event. At point **C**, your emotional Consequence, you feel depressed or self-pitying about this and you want to get rid of this disturbed feeling.

You will recognize this immediately as an example of the A-B-C model of emotional disturbance that we introduced on pages 10–11.

Now, to use REI proceed as follows: as vividly as you can, imagine that you are being severely criticized. You can take an actual example that recently occurred, or you can imagine a future occurrence. As you intensely picture yourself being criticized, let yourself feel really helpless, depressed or self-pitying. Try to get in touch with your emotions of depression or self-pity – don't try to avoid them. Stay with these feelings for a minute or so.

Now, while you keep these unpleasant feelings vividly in your mind, push yourself to make yourself feel *only* disappointed and concerned. If you experience difficulty doing this, try again, and keep trying until you succeed. You can do it! You *can* imagine being severely criticized and make yourself feel *only* concerned and disappointed instead of depressed or self-pitying. Do it!

When you have succeeded and have begun to feel only concerned and disappointed rather than depressed or self-pitying, look closely at what you began to tell yourself at point **B** (your Belief System) to make yourself have these new, healthier feelings. You will find that you probably told yourself something like: 'It's not *awful* to get criticized, but I find it highly inconvenient, unfortunate and rather sad that my parents seemingly have nothing better to do than try to run my life. Although I don't like my parents' constant criticism and wish I could find a way to make them stop, I can definitely stand their criticisms and demands. My life is my own and I can still be happy even if they never change.'

Keep telling yourself these kinds of rBs while you still vividly imagine yourself being criticized and hassled; and continue to *feel* the healthier emotions of disappointment and concern, or regret and displeasure – but not depression or self-pity.

If you spend 10 minutes each day on your Rational-Emotive Imagery (REI), you will get to the point where whenever you recall past episodes of parental demands or criticism, or anticipate future occasions when it might happen, you will tend to feel displeased or disappointed rather than emotionally upset. Then when the day arrives that your parents once more start on you with their criticism and demands, you will be able to handle yourself better. You may feel disappointment and concern over their obnoxious behaviour, but you will avoid upsetting yourself over it.

No matter how poorly you may have reacted to your parents' criticisms in the past, don't put yourself down for it. Accept yourself;

we are all fallible, mistake-making humans. That is our nature, but we can learn from our mistakes and do better in the future. Keep practising Disputing your iBs strongly and vigorously. Practise saying out loud in your rational statements to yourself and do your REI exercise regularly until you easily and automatically begin to feel disappointed, concerned and displeased, rather than depressed and self-pitying when your parents carry on at you with their demands and criticisms.

When you have accomplished these key components of Key Task No. 1, you can proceed with Key Task No. 2.

Key Task No 2: Understanding and accepting your parents with their difficult traits and behaviour

People who act in obnoxious ways, or are difficult to get on with in some aspect, don't just get that way by chance. As we have already pointed out, there are three main reasons for their difficult behaviour: (i) ignorance (ii) emotional disturbance; and (iii) deficiency. Often it is a case of one or more of these reasons. Unfortunately, some difficult parents can exhibit all three! Generally, these three reasons between them cover virtually all kinds of difficult or unacceptable behaviour.

As we have seen, understanding your parents means seeing things from their point of view. Shirley's parents were apparently 'normal' in most other respects; it seems unlikely that they suffered from some kind of organic deficiency or biochemical imbalance. Yet there they were carrying on, dictating to Shirley what she should do or not do. On one occasion, Shirley's mother rang her up to tell her that the new dining-room suite that Shirley and her husband had just bought for their home was a waste of money! Having people around you like that can be a real pain in the neck, but it is worse when they happen to be your parents. They will say they love you, but you could be forgiven for thinking that they have a funny way of showing it.

As a help to understanding your parents, once more try to find out how they themselves were brought up. Was it a very strict type of upbringing? Which of their parents made the major decisions in the house? How was order and discipline maintained? Was much affection displayed within and between members of the family? Were your parents subjected to constant criticism or demands during their formative years, and perhaps later? Maybe your parents grew up with the idea that parents *should* keep an eye on their offspring even after they leave home and get married. They may well have thought that they had a duty to advise you, to criticize your lifestyle, even to

86

override your own decisions if they didn't think your choices were wise.

You can something get a few clues about the way your parents behave towards you now from the way their parents treated them when they were growing up. So make allowances for the influences of family training and the effect of the kind of society your parents were educated and brought up in. You will realize, of course, that your parents' past may well have influenced their thinking to a large degree and contributed towards the way they think and feel now, but the past cannot be held totally responsible for the way they are thinking and feeling today. If the beliefs and attitutes that governed the way your parents behaved in the past are alive and well today, it is because your parents still choose to hold on to these beliefs and attitudes. You may even have identified among them some well-known iBs. However, don't rush in and try to Dispute them. Your primary task is to get on to your parents' wavelength using the method of empathic listening described at some length in previous chapters. Talk to them, but don't criticize them. Listen, and try to make them feel understood. If you succeed, you will improve your chances that they will come to understand you.

That was the task Shirley set herself. Once she had overcome her Low Frustration Tolerance (LFT), she found it easier to assert herself by talking to her parents in the manner suggested above. It is worth bearing in mind that LFT blocks assertive communication, because if you have LFT you tend to be afraid of asserting yourself in case conflict results. 'I'd better not rock the boat, or life will not be easy for me, and I couldn't stand the hassle' is your underlying belief. The trouble with that idea is that by opting for immediate or short-term comfort now, you end up with a good deal more discomfort in the long term. Difficulties don't go away because you shut your eyes to them, and problems tend to multiply.

Shirley persevered with trying to understand her parents' viewpoint, and when she managed eventually to convey to them that she actually appreciated how they felt, they began to look at Shirley through different eyes. It was a new experience for them, something they had never experienced before – feeling really understood by their offspring. If you succeed in making your parents feel understood, you will find them more receptive to your point of view. You are not necessarily trying to get them to agree with it, or you with theirs. The chances are you won't see things the same way; you and they belong to different generations.

The next stage is to accept your parents. This means taking them as they are, and refusing to condemn them for doing things that you find irritating or inconsiderate. For example, the breakthrough for Shirley came when she finally got through to her mother and realized that her mother was afraid that Shirley had left home to get away from her, and that she would lose Shirley altogether unless she kept in constant touch. Shirley's father, seeing how Shirley's mother felt, joined forces and kept up the pressure on Shirley by virtually treating her as if she was still a child living with her parents at home. Shirley realized that her mother was missing her and suffering from the 'empty nest' syndrome. Her mother, it seems, had had a very sheltered childhood and it had taken her a long time to adjust to living without her parents after she had married Shirley's father. Shirley's mother thought that Shirley must feel as strange and insecure as she had done when she left the comfortable certainties of her parents' home and embarked on the uncertainties of married life and starting up a new home. Shirley then realized that her parents' frequent visits and her mother's late-night phone calls, together with both parents' constant criticism and demands to meet their wishes, sprang from a feeling of insecurity. They felt they had to control Shirley's life for fear that they would lose her if they didn't. The more her parents pushed to control her with their criticism and demands, the more defensive Shirley became and the more determined she was to keep her relationship with them at arm's-length; the better Shirley succeeded at this, the more anxious her parents became, and the harder they tried to re-establish control.

After Shirley came to understand her parents better and realized what motivated their behaviour, she relaxed her defensive attitude and began to talk to them in a more friendly manner. Seeing this change of attitude in Shirley, her parents in turn began to open up and to listen to Shirley. She assured them that she was not running away from them, and that she felt the time had come to become more independent. She now had a husband to consider, and Shirley conveyed to her parents that both she and her husband considered that a good relationship with them was possible on the basis of mutual trust and acceptance of one another's rights, and that this was what they both desired. Shirley assured her parents that she loved them, but that she and her husband had got the impression from the way they were being treated that they couldn't be trusted to run their own life and that they needed to be told what to do. 'We now realize you meant well,' Shirley informed her parents. 'We've made mistakes like everyone else, but we're no longer children – and if we are not free to make our own decisions, how are we ever going to learn?'

Of course, not every case of coping with critical and demanding parents in the way outlined in this chapter is guaranteed to produce the results you would like to achieve. Yet even if you understand and accept your parents, but still cannot persuade them to give up their demanding or over-critical ways, you don't have to complain furiously or put yourself down for your failure. Getting angry, depressed or self-pitying won't help you. This doesn't mean that when life seems unfair, or when things don't go the way you would like them to, you should not try to change them. By all means, try! But when you find them unchangeable, don't upset yourself. Practise feeling disappointed, sorry or irritated, not self-pitying or enraged. Accept yourself and others; learn from your past experiences and mistakes, and try to do better in the future. Adopt one of REBT's favourite maxims (first expressed by Reinhold Niebuhr): 'Grant me the courage to change the things I can change, the serenity to accept the things I cannot change, and the wisdom to know the difference.'

Key Task No. 3: Acting in an enlightened self-interested way towards your parents

Having cleared the air between herself and her parents, Shirley set about explaining to them how she and they could help one another in mutually acceptable ways without necessarily infringing each other's individual independence or autonomy. Shirley's husband, Jeff, was also able to go along with that. Initially he resented the constant criticism and demands of Shirley's parents upon them, which he regarded as unwarranted interference in their marriage, and he blamed Shirley for not telling her parents 'to get off our backs!' When he saw the changes that Shirley eventually succeeded in bringing about in her relations with her parents and the better atmosphere that followed, Jeff saw that there were more advantages to be gained from co-operation than by engaging in bitter confrontation.

When you and your parents are on reasonably good speaking terms and can express your views to one another without falling out, or getting into a shouting match when you disagree about something, you can then decide how much contact you are going to have with each other. You may take a short-term view or you can put your ideas into a longer-term framework. Individual circumstances vary. In Shirley's case, she agreed to visit her parents once a week, sometimes accompanied by Jeff, and her parents agreed to visit Shirley once every alternate week. Phone calls would be restricted to just one or two a week, and not after a certain hour at night except in a real emergency. This was rather more often than Shirley would have ideally wished, but she took a long-term view. She and Jeff hoped to start a family one day, and Shirley realized how useful parents can be when they have grandchildren to take out. Grandparents can often be called upon at short notice to look after your children for a couple of hours to allow you to go shopping or keep an appointment, or just to have a couple of uninterrupted hours alone at home with your partner. If you are on really good terms, your parents can sometimes be persuaded to take the children off your hands for three or four days to allow you to have a long weekend away with your partner.

Parents will still want to speak their mind of course. You and they may often disagree, but you can make it clear that you will listen happily to their views if they are expressed in the form of comments or suggestion, but less happily if they come over as criticisms or demands. In other words, you show that you wholeheartedly respect your parents as people with an equal right to their desires and opinions, but you make it clear that you will not permit them to see you as an easy target for exploitation. Adopt an attitude of firm kindness; that means that you don't pamper or baby them. With firm kindness, you act considerately, but you set definite limits as to how far they can impose themselves on you, and you firmly stick to those limits. It's helpful to see things from other people's frames of reference, but never lose sight of your own vital wants and interests.

When you acquire a rational, realistic philosophy of life, you make living your main purpose. You try to make the most of your life by living it to the hilt, by discovering as many interesting and enjoyable things to do as possible, and by setting clear-cut goals and working to achieve them. If you can also help your difficult parents to adopt that philosophy, so much the better.

6

How to Cope with Parents
Who Use Emotional Blackmail

What is emotional blackmail? Putting that question to a group of people selected at random would produce responses like, 'It's when someone you know asks you to do something for them you don't really want to do, but you feel bad about refusing them, so you feel you have to do it so as not to feel mean.' Or, 'A friend or relative will ask you to do something in such a way that you feel like a bad person if you say no.' In other words, emotional blackmail is a ploy adopted by someone to pressurize you into doing something they want you to do by 'making' you feel guilty if you refuse. Since most people prefer 'feeling good' to 'feeling bad', emotional blackmail often works.

Two examples follow of how parents use emotional blackmail to get you to do what they want when it's not what you want, or when it's against your better judgement. Here is the first example:

Your father's birthday is imminent, and he has decided to mark the occasion by formally announcing his retirement from the company he has run as chief executive for many years. In fact, your father handed over the reins to you several months ago, and you have been running the company as chief executive in all but name – a situation that the staff and the shareholders in the company are fully aware of.

Meanwhile, unaware that your father had planned to use his birthday as the occasion to announce his retirement formally, you have made plans of your own for that day. With three friends, you have arranged a week's skiing in Scotland and all the bookings have been made. The particular week you selected was the one most likely, in the opinion of the weather experts, to offer the best snow conditions for skiing.

When your father learns that your planned skiing trip means that you will not be present at his big celebration, he sounds very upset. Patiently, you explain to him why this particular week was selected for your trip. You knew his birthday fell in this particular week, but since he had made no mention to you of his intention to turn the occasion into a retirement party, and since he had not previously made a habit of insisting that you celebrate his birthdays with him, you saw no particular reason to be present at this one.

If you had not made alternative arrangements, you would have been happy to attend his celebration. However, it is now too late to change your plans, and your three friends will be both disappointed and inconvenienced if you cancelled your holiday plans at such short notice. Thus you say to your father, 'Dad, it's *your* special day. You'll have all your old friends and colleagues there. They all know I'm already running things, so it's not as if you really need me there.' Your father replies, 'If you are not present, that will hurt me in a way I will remember to my dying day. If you never do anything for me again as long as I live, just grant me this one request, please, I beg of you!' Consequently, you give in.

Here is the second example:

The group Pink Floyd are back in town and giving a special one-night concert at the giant stadium where they were such a success on their previous visit. This time it's a sell-out, but your boyfriend has somehow managed to get two tickets. You are over the moon with joy. You live with your mother who suffers with asthma, and who is something of a hypochondriac; you tell her your exciting news. 'I'll be out late, Mum, but you'll be all right. I'll get Jenny to look in on you to see that you're OK, and she'll give you your hot drink at bedtime.'

You mother sounds upset. 'You know how I worry about you when you're out late,' she says. 'And when I'm worried, my asthma comes on, and when I can't breathe I get so frightened. It's not fair to put the burden on Jenny. She's a nice girl, but she's not my daughter. It's your duty to look after me, and I can't stand the thought of you being out all those hours late at night. You'll just have to say you can't go, dear. Please, it's for my sake!'

Perhaps you argue with your mother. You may try to reassure her that she'll be all right, as she has been in the past. You so desperately want to go to that concert, but then comes the clincher. Your mother says: 'If you go, I know what's going to happen to me. And you know what the consequences can be when I suffer a really bad attack. I'll leave it to your conscience to decide!' And so you give in.

So who uses emotional blackmail? Just about everybody! Children especially are adept at it. For example, your 11-year-old son tells you that he wants a mountain bike. They're certainly not cheap – a new one can set you back a few hundred pounds. When you demur about spending all that money, your child points out that all his pals have now got mountain bikes and that he is going to be the odd one out. 'People will think we're poor, Dad!' he'll say. Well, you don't want your neighbours to think that, do you! Or your daughter will demand to be allowed to stay out till 10 pm, provided she has finished her homework. 'All the other girls can, Mum. I'm the only one who has to be home so early!' Well, you don't want people to think that you are an over-protective parent, do you! And so you give in.

All these are everyday examples of manipulation by guilt or shame. A more serious example of the use of emotional blackmail is when a rejected suitor threatens to kill himself, or even his beloved, unless she takes him back. This can cause the victim real problems, for no one can be sure whether or not the threat will be carried out. Quite often it isn't carried out, but when the blackmailer is in such an emotionally disturbed state of mind, who can be sure?

The trouble is that the more often you give in to emotional blackmail, the more often you will find it used against you. People, including children, learn to interact with others in ways that experience shows works most easily. If, for example, encouraging others to feel guilty produces the desired result, then the manipulator will use guilt. Or it might be shame, fear or embarrassment. Whatever is found to work most easily will be employed.

We provided these examples of manipulation by guilt or shame to bring out the essence of emotional blackmail. From this point on, we will focus our attention on the more serious consequences of emotional blackmail when parents use it to control the lives, or some aspect of the lives, of their adult offspring. The main point to bear in mind is that emotional blackmail has one purpose: control of someone else's behaviour. When emotional blackmail is used against you, the user aims to exploit your ability to feel guilt or shame for his or her own ends. The good news is that you can't be manipulated without your permission. By means of an example, we will show you how to cope with emotional blackmail and how to deal with your own feelings that arise in the process. You will also see the negative effects that follow when emotional blackmail is not resisted and effectively dealt with.

The case of Mark and Shareena

Mark was a young man of 25. Born in England of English parents, he held an MSc degree in science and worked as an analytical chemist for a well-known drug company. Of presentable appearance, Mark was popular with his colleagues and was generally easy to get on with.

Shareena was 21, and worked as a private secretary to the head of the department where Mark was employed. Shareena had been born in the

Punjab, and had come to England with her parents when she was a baby. Brought up in England, Shareena had done well at school and, after gaining several secretarial qualifications had obtained her present job as private secretary to Dr Cama, who headed the department where Mark worked. Mark and Shareena were attracted to each other from the beginning and were soon dating on a regular basis. It was not long before they realized they were in love, and they decided to get engaged.

Unfortunately, the news of their engagement did not go down well with Shareena's parents. They were upset that their daughter had decided to marry an Englishman, and they considered it their parental duty to stop the proposed marriage from going ahead. Shareena's father had already earmarked a wealthy young bachelor with close links to Shareena's own family as a suitable husband for Shareena, and he didn't want his plans disrupted by his daughter's apparently wayward infatuation for Mark. The rest of Shareena's family, with the exception of her younger sister, were agreed that this was the right thing to do. Shareena's parents resolved to persuade her to break off her engagement to Mark.

Shareena was shocked and dismayed. Although the possibility of parental interference in her choice of marital partner had occurred to her, she had not taken it too seriously. After all, this was England in the last decade of the twentieth century. People here freely chose who *they* wanted to marry, and not some comparative stranger selected for them by parents or guardians. Surely her parents who had adapted so well to Western customs and behaviour, and who were perfectly conversant with how young people here went about choosing their partners, would have the sense to know that this was the way their own daughter would choose when the time came for her to make up her mind? Shareena decided to inform her parents that her mind was made up, and that there was no way that she would break her engagement to Mark.

At this point, Shareena really believed that she could reason with her parents and persuade them to accept her decision to marry Mark. However, she soon found to her dismay that her perception of her parents was wrong.

Dealing with emotional blackmail

Mind control is what many parents try to achieve over their children's thinking. It then becomes easier to get their offspring to behave in ways that are acceptable to the parents. Shareena's parents set about changing the way their daughter thought about marriage and the effect that her marriage to an Englishman would have on her relationship with her parents, and the community into which she had been born, if she went ahead with her plans to marry Mark.

First, Shareena's parents talked long and hard with her about her family history, about her people's traditions and beliefs that went back thousands of years. Surely she hadn't forgotten those ancient teachings she had learnt as a child and that her parents and forebears had learnt and practised over the centuries? As Shareena's parents explained to her, 'Our family, our people, have always done things this way. We have a noble heritage and we are proud of our history. Think of all those cultural values that have been handed down to us from the past to preserve and practise. They have stood the test of time. Compare them with the "here-today-gone-tomorrow" standards that you see all around you today. Do you really think Western society can teach us anything of value compared to the priceless heritage with which we have been endowed? Who are you to go against centuries of tradition and teaching? What makes *you* think you know better than the sages who gave us our religion, our philosophy, our learning?'

When Shareena protested that Mark was a nice man and that her parents would like him, they replied that Mark's character had nothing to do with it. 'He is not of our people,' explained her father, 'and he never will be. You might as well forget him, because you will marry who we tell you to marry, and not some English boy who has caught your fancy!'

In tears, Shareena implored her father to accept that she loved Mark and that she would never marry anyone else, especially someone she didn't love. It was to no avail. When her father realized that Shareena was determined to stick to her decision to marry Mark, he told her, 'In that case, neither I, nor any other member of this family, will ever speak to you again! Nor will anyone in our community ever speak to you or have anything to do with you. You will be seen as a disgrace to yourself, to me, to all your family, and to all your people who have nurtured you and stood by you all these years. From the moment you leave this house to go to your Englishman, you will no longer be my daughter. You will be nothing! You have brought nothing but shame upon this house and upon this community of which you are a part. Do you understand me? Go against me and you will lose your family, you will lose everything!'

Faced with this ultimatum, Shareena did nothing but sob and sob until she felt she had cried her heart out. She loved Mark, but she also loved her family. 'Why do they have to treat me like this?' she sobbed. 'I have been made to feel I am a horrible person, just because I love someone they don't approve of. What is wrong with him anyway? Nothing! They aren't even giving him a chance! They don't want to know him just because he isn't a member of our community. I can't bear it!' Shareena then cried herself to sleep in sheer exhaustion.

Now let's see how Shareena could deal with the situation confronting her. Her father, with the support of his family, is trying to blackmail Shareena emotionally into giving up the man she loves and wants to marry. He has made it clear to her that if she goes against his wishes, she loses everything. She will be regarded as a pariah, shunned by all those she loved and who she thought loved her. Shareena, understandably, is upset. She will not go back on her decision to marry Mark. Her problem now is to discover how she can deal with the emotional impact of being expelled from the family that she still loves. Her immediate task is to get herself into the right frame of mind where she can take a realistic look at her situation, and then decide what attitude she can sensibly take towards her family so as to mimimize the impact of her expulsion and to avoid seeing herself in a self-pitying light. This is Shareena's first Key Task, to which we now devote our attention.

Key Task No. 1: Getting yourself into a healthy frame of mind emotionally

Bear in mind that Shareena's decision will lead to her instant dismissal from her family as soon as they know for sure that she intends going against her parents' wishes. Her fiancé, Mark, is standing by her and has assured her that their plans to marry still stand, but he is leaving the decision to leave, or stay, entirely with Shareena. He realizes that Shareena is under enough stress already as a result of the pressure and threats from her parents, and that any pressure from him would be counterproductive. He believes that she will stand by her decision to marry him and resist the pressure from her parents to give him up.

Shareena's immediate task is to challenge the belief (that she now holds) that she will be a horrible or worthless person if her family cast her out. Her belief about her situation is:

- 'I absolutely must not lose the love and approval of my family and other significant or important people in my community, or else I will rate as a worthless person – and I can't bear that!'

Disputing Shareena's iBs

Now let's examine this belief to see whether it can stand up to critical examination. Being cut off by one's family, especially in the circumstances described above, can be a serious matter – especially for a young adult – and we are not attempting to minimize it. However, if the matter can be viewed realistically and in the context of a young adult woman with virtually her whole life in front of her, it can be realized that a family calamity is not necessarily a personal catastrophe. So let's apply the criteria of rationality to Shareena's belief that she is a worthless person without her parents' love and approval.

(a) *Is this belief logical?* No. Shareena obviously does not want to lose the love and approval of her family, but it doesn't logically follow that she absolutely must not.

Even if she does lose the love and approval of certain people, it does not logically follow that she will rate as a worthless person. That may be the view of some people, even of Shareena herself, but it is only an arbitrary definition that her personal worth depends on whether certain people love and approve of her.

Nor does it logically follow that if her parents and significant others were to withdraw their love and approval of Shareena, that she couldn't possibly bear the loss. All she can logically conclude from losing the love of certain people is that the behaviour of those people towards her is likely to change.

(b) *Is this belief consistent with reality?* If there were some law of the universe that said that Shareena absolutely must not lose the love and approval of certain people who are important to her, then she wouldn't. Since no such law exists, Shareena's demand makes no sense.

Next, how can losing certain people's love and approval make one a worthless person? As you will know by now, you cannot legitimately rate a person as good or bad. A person is an ongoing entity comprised of many traits, abilities and characteristics that change over the individual's lifetime.

Moreover, this belief is a gross over-generalization because it takes one aspect of Shareena – her desire to marry her English fiancé – and identifies the entire personhood of Shareena with that one aspect. The entire personality of Shareena is shrunk down to just one thing: her desire to marry Mark! And because that is defined as totally bad, she herself becomes totally bad or worthless. To term this belief unrealistic is something of an understatement!

Shareena's belief that she 'can't bear' losing the love and approval of people who are important to her is not true. There are many unpleasant, painful things in life you would prefer not to bear, but there is no evidence that they will lead to your instant demise.

(c) *Will this belief help Shareena to achieve her goals?* That would appear to be very unlikely. Once you take on board the absurd notion that you lose all of your worth as a human being, meaning that you are of no value whatever to yourself, you will certainly not be motivated to strive for what you want out of life. For what would be the point? If you cease to have any value to yourself, what is the point of living?

If you refer back to page 51, you will see that Shareena is holding Major Irrational Belief No. 1. She needs to Dispute this vigorously, and replace it with the following rational alternative beliefs.

Shareena's rational alternative beliefs

- 'While I strongly prefer to continue to receive love and approval from my parents and other significant people in my community, there is no reason why they must do as I wish. They respond to what goes on in their heads and not to what goes on in mine. Life must go on, and I accept myself as a person with a right to live and enjoy my life as I choose, so long as I do not gratuitously interfere with the rights of others to live as they choose. If I am rejected by my family and community, that will be quite unfortunate and disadvantageous for me in several ways, but I can obviously bear it – although I'll never like it. I will be happy to respond at any time to genuine moves by my family to restore communications with me. But if it is not to be, that will be too bad, but hardly the end of the world.'

Shareena's new 'healthy negative feelings'

As a consequence of acquiring a more rational view of her situation, Shareena's changed way of thinking will lead her to feel differently about her rejection by her family. She certainly won't feel happy about it – she neither wanted nor expected such an outcome. Shareena had hoped that her decision to marry Mark would be welcomed by her family, and that eventually Mark would be accepted as a member of it. Unfortunately, Shareena's family had different ideas.

Shareena's more rational beliefs about her family's rejection of her would lead her to feel extremely sad and disappointed, but not desperately miserable and totally worthless. She realizes that losing her family is a misfortune, but that she doesn't have to lose herself. She can accept herself with the right to make her own life choices, even if her family does not accept that.

Once Shareena is fully convinced that she would prefer to have her parents on her side as she prepares for her marriage to Mark, but that she doesn't *have* to have their approval, she can go ahead, prepared to pay the price of losing her family, if that is the way it has to be. There is always a price to pay. There is rarely such a thing as something for nothing. The greater the happiness you wish to achieve, the greater the price you must pay to achieve it. It's your responsibility to decide how great a price you are willing to pay, and it is to your advantage to decide on that price before you take action. If you were in Shareena's position, or facing a similar kind of problem with your own family, you might decide that losing your family was too high a price to pay. That is why it is so important to make these decisions when you are thinking clearly and rationally. When you are emotionally upset, you cannot think rationally – that is, logically, realistically, and able to balance the pros and cons of a difficult situation as it is, and not as you think it ought to be, or would like it to be.

Key Task No. 2: Understanding and accepting your parents with their difficult traits and behaviours

If you have attentively read the preceding chapters, you should have acquired some understanding of what it means to understand and accept your parents. Clearly, if your parents carry out their threats to disown you, or refuse to speak to you ever again, you won't even get the chance to employ those communication skills and empathic listening skills we have been trying to teach you throughout this book! However, although we see no point in repeating what we said under this paragraph heading in the preceding chapters, a few additional points seem worth making. Then, if your parents one day relent and indicate that they want to get back on speaking terms with you again, at least you will be prepared to respond appropriately.

Understanding your parents means seeing things from their point of view, but it takes on a special importance when these parents are members of an ethnic minority. If your parents have threatened to cut off all contact with you, as was the case with Shareena, it is not because they are just being vindictive or bloody-minded. They probably feel very upset at losing you. In Shareena's case, her decision to go ahead with her plans to marry her English fiancé contributed to the sense of shame experienced by her parents at what they saw as their failure to maintain important family and cultural traditions. You should understand that throughout history practically every ethnic or religious minority has done its best to preserve its cultural and religious customs and traditions by maintaining a certain distance from itself and the customs, beliefs and values of the society in which the minority group finds itself. It is the only way in which it can preserve its cultural identity and ensure its survival and continuity. If the younger members of the group are allowed to marry 'outsiders', or are even allowed to import too many of the host society's values, it won't be too many generations before the minority group will have virtually disappeared in all but name. Expulsion from the group is essentially a measure of self-preservation. It is a defence against the gradual dilution of the minority group's identity.

If you happen to have a similar problem to Shareena's, don't raise your hopes too high of persuading your parents to accept you back. In all probability, they are deeply upset at expelling you. They still love you, but the maintenance of family and cultural traditions and the homogeneity of the community to which they belong, and always will belong, takes precedence over personal desires. If an exception were to be made in your case, others would follow sooner or later. The choice for you is almost certainly this: stay – or stay away for ever. Hence, you would be wise to think through thoroughly the foreseeable consequences of each choice to ensure that your final decision is the one you feel you can comfortably live with.

Not all cases of parental pressure via emotional blackmail will be as dramatic as the one described. You may find that if you stick to your guns and refuse to allow yourself to be manipulated by fear, guilt or shame, that your parents will relent and allow some degree of communication to be re-established. You will then have the opportunity to use the communication skills outlined in our previous chapters to good effect. As we have seen, accepting your parents means taking them as they are, acknowledging that they have the right to make whatever decisions they consider are right for them in the circumstances, and refusing to condemn them for making decisions that you consider hurtful and sad. Remember, your parents may have felt they had little choice in the matter. If you have to leave them and the community in which you were brought up and were reasonably happy, harbouring resentment against them will do you no good.

Try not to 'personalize' their behaviour. In less dramatic examples of emotional blackmail, you would do well to remember that as a result of their own tendencies to think irrationally and to behave negatively, parents' actions may strike you as unnecessarily inconsiderate, provocative or stupid, but because of their own unresolved problems they will continue to drive themselves to act in stupid and self-defeating ways. By refusing to allow your feelings to be manipulated and by showing that you understand and accept them, you may make some headway towards persuading them to give up their manipulative ploys and to treat you in a more considerate manner.

If your efforts are to no avail and your parents' manipulative behaviour seems to be unchangeable, practise feeling disappointed, sorry or displeased. Resentment or self-pity will get you nowhere and may well make things worse; don't try to get close to your parents. Wait until you see signs that they are prepared to treat your fairly and honestly, then respond in kind.

Key Task No. 3: Acting in an enlightened self-interested way towards your parents

Once you have made what you truly believe to be the decision that is in your best interests, stick to it! Don't allow yourself to be influenced or manipulated by the unsolicited opinions of others. You are an adult person; no other living person has the right to decide what is right or wrong for you. Remember, 'selfishness' is not the issue; you have but one life to live. If you are aware of what you are doing and why you are doing it, it makes sense to do everything within your power to make your life as pleasant and fulfilling as you can. That is what enlightened self-interest means: acting in your own best interests at least most of the time.

Now let's get back to Shareena again. In deciding to marry her fiancé, Mark, she was acting in what she thought would be in her long-term best interests. The price Shareena paid for her courageous decision was ostracism by her family. Does that mean that Shareena has to abandon her religion and try to forget all those values she acquired during her upbringing by her parents? Not at all! Remember, Shareena still loves her parents in spite of their decision to sever contact with her. She understands why they acted as they did, and she knows how much their decision to abandon her must have hurt them. For the time being, at least, she and her parents will have no contact. But Shareena, while regretting this situation, does not see it as being in her best interests to abandon her parents emotionally by trying to forget all that they meant to her. She is not trying to become a different person. Shareena chose Mark because she loved him; and Mark, for his part, loves Shareena as she is. Neither wants to change the other. All they both want is to continue being the two people they are, and to build a life for themselves as a married couple. If Shareena, out of spite, began to act and behave in ways uncharacteristic of her and deliberately at variance with the way she had been brought up, in order to affront her family, she would only be defeating herself. When word eventually got round to Shareena's parents about the way she was carrying on, her parents would feel even more upset, and take this latest manifestation of their daughter's waywardness as justification for their decision to eject her from her family and community.

As we have stated, it is not in your best interests needlessly to antagonize people who mean something to you. If you think there is even a small chance of bringing about a better relationship between yourself and your parents, it may make sense to try for some kind of rapprochement. This might occur eventually if you show by your behaviour that you bear your parents no animosity, and that you are not trying to upset them.

Nothing is necesarily permanent about relationships. Relationships are made, broken and re-made by innumerable individuals every day. Even when a relationship appears to have irretrievably ended, it can happen sometimes that the players involved have second thoughts. Then they may take steps to restore communication, and perhaps end up by getting back together again. But remember, there are no guarantees!

Now, while we are on the subject of acting in an enlightened self-interested way, let's note a number of relevant points it will pay you to keep in mind:

• Learning from experience helps to prepare you for long-term success as you strive to reach your goals. While you are enduring the bumps, bruises and hassles that life constantly throws in your way, there is a free hand-out with each situation. It's called an 'educational experience'. If you extract the lesson to be learned from it, you will be better prepared the next time round to deal with a similar situation. We would admit that some learning experiences can be very hard indeed, but these, at least, are the kind you are unlikely to forget.

• Everything in life has a price is another key fact of existence. If you didn't know it already, not only does everything in life that you value and desire carry a price tag, but the price you pay can take many forms. Whatever adds pleasure to your existence – be it love, friendship, fame, money, or the freedom to come and go as you please – must be paid for. The payment may take the form of money, time, energy, patience, hard work, discomfort or practically anything else. In Shareena's case, she paid the price of losing her family for the foreseeable future, and maybe for ever. Whatever it is, pay the price and get it over with. Don't attempt to buy what you want on the 'instalment plan'. Short-term solutions – such as buying time or compromising on matters of principle in the hope of avoiding the ultimate payment – often make the long-term solutions that much harder to reach, as well as being much more costly. If you opt for the easy way out, you'll find yourself stuck in the 'Comfort Trap' (For advice on this issue, see our book *Beating the Comfort Trap*, Sheldon Press, 1993.)

• Acquiring self-discipline is a basic necessity if you really want to live your life in an enlightened self-interested way, and to reap the benefits of doing so. Dispense with typical rationalizations that you will solve a given problem later. 'Later' never seems to come! And don't assume that the problem will just go away if you wait long enough. Is it really worth giving up years and years of precious time to avoid a tough confrontation? The sooner you take the time and expend the necessary effort to work out long-term, permanent solutions now, the more pleasurable your life will become. Let others cling to their cosy niches. Not much will go wrong for them, but not much will happen either. Be adventurous, take sensible risks, and begin paying the price in full as soon as possible.

Whatever your goals may be, conscious, self-disciplined, rationally directed effort will get you there sooner than anything else. Being fully responsible for realizing your desires and goals is what self-discipline is all about. We can assure you that no one else is going to do the job of looking after your vital interests as well as you yourself.

• Acquiring a realistic perspective is another useful tool in your intellectual kitbag if, like Shareena, you find yourself being ostracized by members of your family and/or ethnic group. It's a pain when people you knew and loved turn against you because you no longer subscribe to their views on how you should conduct your life, but a 'pain' relative to what? Is it as bad as being permanently unemployed when you'd give anything for a job? Is it as bad as being paralysed by a stroke, or being diagnosed as having a terminal cancer? A good way of avoiding the tendency to 'awfulize' and to feel sorry for yourself when the going gets tough is to remind yourself that no matter how bad things may seem now, they could always get worse.

You may well get called uncomplimentary names when you get expelled from a family or community, or indeed from any kind of group. The idea is to 'shame' you because you had the nerve to stand up for what you believed was the right thing to do against all those self-appointed moralists, experts or guardians whose aim it is to maintain the status quo. Does it really matter to you if people, particularly those who advocate political or religious doctrines, moral codes or values that you consider out of date and unrealistic, tongue-lash you with names? They're only words, and they cannot hurt you unless you let them. So don't allow yourself to be hurt or intimidated by words, and don't waste your time explaining yourself to name-callers. Ignore them and continue to look after your own interests. Taking full responsibility for your own decisions is a sign of maturity. Equally, do not allow people to do things for you that they really would rather not do. It may sometimes pay you to 'look a gifthorse in the mouth' if you have reason to believe that receiving a 'gift' from someone is going to be used later by the giver as a bargaining unit to get something out of you.

• 'Is it worth going back?' is a question that may arise if your parents, realizing that their emotional blackmailing tactics don't work, suggest resuming some kind of closer relationship with you. If your original problem was similar to Shareena's, it is unlikely that you will be confronted with this decision. If your parents were the more common variety of manipulators with no special cultural or religious axe to grind, you can consider each case on its merits.

Try to find out why your parents are now trying to change. Is it genuine, and is it likely to last? Or is it just another ploy to get round you? Use the skills you learned earlier under Key Task No. 2 to test them out. Let them know that you will not respond to manipulation, but that you will at least consider any reasonable proposition that is put to you fairly and squarely.

Decide how much time or work will be involved and whether the gain is likely to be worth the time and effort. Does it entail any sacrifice of your own primary interests? In Shareena's case, there might be a possibility of her being taken back by her parents provided she were to leave Mark. She would be very unlikely to consider any such thing, but it can, and does, happen.

If you see advantages to be gained by getting back with your parents, what is being asked of you in return? What are the rules or conditions? It is important to be very clear in your mind about what your primary interests are; and, before you decide anything, to distinguish your primary interests from your secondary interests. The bottom line is, as always, the price you are being asked to pay, and in what 'currency'.

Finally, if after rational analysis you take what for you seems the right decision at the time, but which later and more accurate information convinces you was the wrong decision by your standards, do not in any way allow yourself to feel guilty. Guilt, as we have consistently reiterated throughout this book, is never the solution. If it is appropriate, make the necessary apologies in a head-up, straightforward manner. You are a mistake-prone animal like everyone else. The practical solution to your error? Learn from your experience, remember the lesson learned, then forget about your mistake and concentrate on not repeating it the next time around. Don't put yourself down for having made a bad decision.

Have the courage of your convictions!

Shareena showed that she had the courage of her convictions by standing by her decision and following it up without knowing for sure whether her decision was right or wrong. She has not regretted her decision to marry Mark, although she does miss her family. That was to be expected. From time to time, Shareena receives secret snippets of information from her younger sister telling her what is happening in her family circle. Shareena is happy to know that her parents miss her and are sorry to lose her, but so far they are sticking to their decision to have nothing whatever to do with her. That, too, was to be expected. Perhaps in time Shareena's parents will change their mind, especially if they realize that their daughter is doing well and has not suffered the bad consequences that some members of her community had predicted. By showing that she bears no grudges and has no animosity towards her family, Shareena has made it possible for some kind of reconciliation to take place should her family one day decide to take the initiative to bring it about.

You don't need certainty!

No one knows what the future will bring; no one knows for certain whether important decisions made now will turn out for the best in the long run. You make the best decision in the light of the information and knowledge you have at the time about the possible consequences, but you can't be certain. If you demand that you wait until you are certain of the outcome before you take a decision, you'll wait for ever! Trying to live your life fully does involve taking reasonable risks, of experimentally determining what it is you like and dislike, and then doing what you judge to be in your best long-term interests, while accepting that you live in a world of probability and chance.

Afterword

The six chapters in this book have taken as their themes typical examples of parental behaviour that adult children find difficult to cope with. The examples selected enabled us to set forth certain principles that, when properly understood, can be applied to the resolution of practically any kind of difficult parental behaviour that you, as an adult, may be confronted with. So even if your parents present you with a particular problem that does not fit neatly into any of the categories of difficult parental behaviour covered in these six chapters, you can still use the principles and methods described throughout the book to tackle your own particular problem.

Understanding the principles and methods outlined in each chapter is an essential prerequisite to taking effective action to deal with the kind of problems you may experience when trying to cope with difficult parents. However, as we have reiterated, acquiring *insight* into the nature of these problems is not in itself enough to resolve them. Let us explain why this is so.

Intellectual insight alone is not enough

Once you have covered the REBT concepts and techniques outlined in each chapter, it is easy to fall into the trap of thinking that once you have read and understood them, no further action is required. The basic principles of REBT are not difficult to grasp, and any reasonably intelligent and motivated person can understand them if willing to devote a little time and effort to the task. However, merely understanding what we are teaching is not enough. Resistance to new ideas is enormous. Even if you find our advocacy of rational ways of thinking entirely convincing, and are trying hard to acquire them, you are going to have to practise and work tenaciously at uprooting your previous, much longer held, iBs and replacing them with rational alternative beliefs, before you find yourself *habitually* thinking along rational lines and staying emotionally healthy. For many years you have been used to thinking along irrational lines, so your old ideas are not just going to curl up and die overnight because you realize that they are no longer tenable! It is when you look at the emotional side of life – at the emotional dramas and traumas, the rampant superstition, and the tragedies that often follow over-emotionalized, over-dramaticized and exaggerated thinking – that you realize the immense influence of iBs in creating and sustaining human misery. Let's face it, the vast majority of human beings find it difficult to change their irrational behaviour even when they 'know' perfectly well that they are behaving stupidly and against their best interests, and even when they acquire some insight into the causes of their self-defeating behaviour. That is why we continually stress the need for hard work and practice if you are going to acquire a more rational outlook on life.

If trying to cope with difficult parents is a major problem for you as you strive to make the most of your own limited time on this planet, it is imperative that you acquire the right frame of mind before you tackle the problem, in order to have a reasonable hope of successfully resolving it. If you are emotionally disturbed yourself, how can you expect to cope with the disturbed feelings and behaviour of others – especially the kind you can come up against with difficult parents? This, of course, underlines the central importance of accomplishing Key Task No. 1 (Getting yourself into a healthy frame of mind emotionally). Acquiring a rational philosophy and practising it puts you in the right frame of mind; it puts you in the driving seat, as it were. Then, equipped with the skills and insights you will derive from carrying out Key Task No. 2 (Understanding and accepting your parents, with their difficult traits and behaviour), you will have the 'know-how' and the 'emotional muscle' you need to steer a course through the 'minefields' that often impede the development of a healthier relationship with your parents. Once you've reached that point, completing Key Task No. 3 (Acting in an enlightened self-interested way towards your parents) will provide you with your bearings as you chart the kind of relationship with your parents you are hoping to achieve.

A few tips

Here are a few tips to help you build on your intellectual insight.

- To act as a constant reminder to yourself, type or write the three REBT Insights on a postcard and keep it in your wallet or handbag. Make a point of looking at your card and reading these REBT Insights at least once a day.

- Re-read Chapter 1 several times until you know and fully understand it. Pay particular attention to the A–B–C model of emotional disturbance and the criteria of rationality, then test your understanding of the material by seeing if you can explain it correctly to somebody who knows nothing about it. To explain a subject correctly to someone else is a measure of how well you yourself understand it!

- Be clear in your own mind *why* iBs cannot be accepted as true. See how many variants of the three Major Irrational Beliefs you can come up with, and keep a handy note of them for frequent reference (on another card, like the one you used for recording the three REBT Insights). Look at them often! Keep looking for your 'absolutistic' demands upon yourself, your parents, and the world in general – the *shoulds*, *oughts* and *musts*. When you find them, vigorously Dispute them until you no longer believe them, and replace them with flexible, non-dogmatic desires and preferences. And while you are at it, don't forget to combat your old tendencies to 'awfulize' and 'catastrophize' about your life situation when the world doesn't immediately grant you what you demand it must, or when your 'difficult' parents still refuse to change their ways and insist on carrying on as they always have, in spite of your noble efforts to persuade them otherwise.

- Be sure you understand *why* rBs will lead you to experience healthier feelings, and help to bring you better results in your personal relationships.

- Make sure that you know and appreciate the distinction we frequently make between 'healthy negative feelings' and 'unhealthy negative feelings', and why the difference is important. Make sure that you know how to change unhealthy negative feelings to healthier feelings by identifying and disputing the iBs underlying the unhealthy negative feelings.

- Practise using Rational-Emotive Imagery (REI) to prepare yourself in advance to cope with difficult situations involving your parents that you anticipate could trigger off unhealthy negative feelings such as anxiety, anger, shame or embarrassment. Work at your REI exercises until you are able to replace these unhealthy negative feelings with healthy negative alternative feelings – such as concern, annoyance or displeasure, and regret.

Beware of over-generalizations and exaggerations!

These represent forms of extremism, as well as being fairly typical examples of irrational thinking. For example, you don't just conclude that your parents acted in a selfish and uncaring manner when they failed to carry out a promise they made to you the other day, and as a consequence put you to needless expense; no, you go beyond the facts and easily conclude that they will *always* be selfish and uncaring. Or, if it would cause you a certain amount of inconvenience if a certain event were to occur, such as having one or both of your parents to live with you and be looked after for an indefinite period, you easily convince yourself that it will be a terrible catastrophe if it does occur.

As you work through Key Task No. 2 (Understanding and accepting your parents with their difficult traits and behaviour), you may find it helpful to make allowances for your parents' tendencies to think in these ways, and to look out for and avoid similar instances of exaggerated 'all-or-nothing' thinking on your part.

What to do when you slip back

It's a fairly common experience when learning something new to find yourself slipping back. Let's say you seem to be making progress towards improving your relationship with your parents. You have accomplished the Three Key Tasks, and then you repeat some error you thought you had previously got rid of.

For example, suppose you have in fact been making progress at getting along with your parents instead of being continually at loggerheads with them as you were at one time. One day you go to visit them, intending to discuss a matter that had been bothering you. Somehow, your parents misread your intentions and begin to argue with you; they make accusations against you that you consider grossly unfair. Before you know it, a shouting match is taking place, just like in the old days, and you abruptly depart, seething with indignation. Then when you have cooled down, you savagely berate yourself for having lost your temper. Losing your temper has put your improved relationship with your parents back to where it was in the bad old days when you and they were hardly on speaking terms.

It does you no good to put yourself down and to feel ashamed or angry with yourself if, for example, you have lost your temper. Accept it as normal, as the sort of mistake humans make from time to time. Do you recall our frequent emphasis on the importance of self-acceptance, and of accepting other people as well as yourself as fallible human beings who frequently make mistakes because that is our nature? That should give you your clue as to what to do next. What you do is go back to basics, and work harder and harder on your iBs by Disputing them. Don't waste energy by putting yourself down for failing. The secret is to practise going over and over again the three Major Irrational Beliefs, the three REBT Insights, the A–B–C model of emotional disturbance and the various worked examples of Disputing iBs, using the variety of techniques we have outlined throughout the text. These are the fundamentals; they are also the foundation stones on which your Three Key Tasks are built.

Don't forget the importance of *acting* against your iBs until you become comfortable doing things you previously were afraid to try. Action is a great way of counterattacking anxiety-producing ideas. For example, are you afraid of how your parents will react when you tell them that you want to leave home and start living on your own? Or, if you want your parents to spend more time with you and to show you and your child a bit more affection, are you afraid to approach and ask them for fear of being rejected or laughed at? An effective way to overcome any kind of anxiety is to *do* what you are irrationally afraid of doing, and at the same time, as you force yourself to act, challenge and question the nonsensical assumptions – the iBs – you are telling yourself to make yourself anxious or ashamed. Monitor your progress, and convince yourself that you really can make headway if you work at it.

To end on a high note, we re-emphasize that one of the hallmarks of an emotionally healthy human being is to become creatively absorbed in some long-range goal or project. We have already supplied you with the tools you will need to achieve that in the form of the various REBT thinking and feeling techniques and communication skills we have taught in this book. We believe that these, together with those you will find in our other books published by Sheldon Press, will be of considerable help to you in coping successfully with 'difficult' parents, and, in addition, will help you to achieve whatever other goals in life you have set yourself.

To remain emotionally healthy and to direct your own life confidently, keep practising these REBT techniques on a daily basis until they become truly established as an integral part of your psychological make-up. You will benefit not only yourself, but also your loved ones – and not least, perhaps, even your 'difficult' parents!

We wish you every success!

Index